THRIVING ON PLANTS

A Journey to Health Through Veganism

Thriving on Plants: A Journey to Health and Wholeness
Copyright © 2025 by Dr. Sandra Michael-Johnson

All rights reserved. No part of this publication may be reproduced, distributed, or transmitted in any form or by any means, including photocopying, recording, or other electronic or mechanical methods, without the prior written permission of the author, except in the case of brief quotations used in critical reviews and other noncommercial uses permitted by copyright law.

For permission requests, please contact:
Dr. Sandra Michael-Johnson @ info@smjbsolutions.com

ISBN: 979-8-9937371-0-2
Cover Design: Ushan Creations
Author Photo: Dr. Sandra Michael-Johnson
Printed in the United States of America

First Edition, 2025

Preface

When I first began this journey, I was not looking for a trend or a quick fix. I was looking for healing. As the owner of national healthcare agencies, I have witnessed firsthand the devastating effects of chronic illness on individuals, families, and communities. Yet, despite my professional expertise, I found myself facing my own health scare. Fatigue had become my constant companion, and a brush with hypertension forced me to pause and reflect.

I realized that to continue serving others, I first needed to serve myself. To lead, I had to live the example I wanted for my patients, my community, and my family. This realization became the doorway to my plant-based journey.

Transitioning to a vegan lifestyle has been more than a dietary shift; it has been a transformation of body, mind, and spirit. I discovered energy, clarity, and balance I never thought possible. Most importantly, I discovered a renewed sense of purpose: to share not only the science of plant-based living but also the humanity of it—the everyday struggles, the triumphs, and the deep joy that comes from nourishing oneself in alignment with wellness.

This book is not just about food. It is about freedom—freedom from fatigue, from preventable illness, from cycles of disconnection from our bodies. It is my story, but it is also an invitation for you to begin your own.

May these pages encourage you, support you, and remind you that you are capable of lasting, life-giving change.

With gratitude,

Dr. Sandra Michael-Johnson

Acknowledgments

I would like to express my deepest gratitude to my family and loved ones, who supported me with patience and encouragement throughout this journey.

To my colleagues and community in healthcare, thank you for inspiring me to always seek better ways to heal and thrive.

To the many individuals who have shared their own stories of resilience and transformation, you have reminded me that this work matters and that every journey can inspire another.

And to all readers of this book—thank you for taking this step toward a healthier, more compassionate life. May your journey be filled with strength, healing, and joy.

With gratitude,

Dr. Sandra Michael-Johnson

Dedication

To my family, whose love has been my foundation.
To those who have faced health challenges with courage and determination.
And to every reader ready to take this step toward healing and wholeness this book is for you.

Thriving on Plants: A Health-First Guide to Going Vegan

- The rise of plant-based eating
- Why health is a driving motivator
- Dispelling myths about veganism

Chapter 1: Why Go Vegan for Health?

- Scientific evidence on plant-based diets
- Reduced risk of heart disease, diabetes, and cancer
- Longevity and vitality

Chapter 2: Understanding Nutrition, the Vegan Way

- Macronutrients: proteins, fats, carbohydrates
- Micronutrients: vitamins and minerals
- Common concerns (B12, iron, calcium, omega-3s, protein)

Chapter 3: Preparing for the Transition

- Assessing your current diet
- Setting health goals
- The mindset shift: addition vs. restriction

Chapter 4: Stocking Your Vegan Kitchen

- Pantry essentials (grains, beans, nuts, seeds)
- Fresh produce staples
- Smart swaps for everyday meals

Chapter 5: The First 30 Days

- Step-by-step transition plan
- Sample meal ideas

- How to handle cravings

Chapter 6: Eating Out & Social Life

- Navigating restaurants
- Traveling vegan
- Dealing with friends and family

Chapter 7: Fitness and Energy on Plants

- Building muscle on a vegan diet
- Energy for endurance and recovery
- Real-life athlete examples

Chapter 8: Common Challenges and How to Overcome Them

- Digestive adjustments
- Label reading and hidden animal products
- Dealing with setbacks

Chapter 9: The Long-Term Health Benefits

- Disease prevention in detail
- Healthy aging and mental clarity
- The link between gut health and immunity

Chapter 10: Living Vibrantly as a Vegan

- Finding community
- Sustainable lifestyle choices
- Embracing abundance

Chapter 11: Plant-based Lifestyle

- Learning the science of plant-based health
- Navigating your first 30 days
- Finding a deeper meaning

Chapter 12: Conclusion

- Thriving, not just surviving
- Your health as an investment
- Inspiration for the lifelong journey

The Connection Between Veganism and Mental Health

In addition to its physical and environmental benefits, adopting a vegan lifestyle can have a profound impact on mental and emotional well-being. What we eat not only fuels our bodies it nourishes our minds, shapes our moods, and influences how we respond to stress.

Nourishing the Brain Naturally

A whole-food, plant-based diet is rich in antioxidants, vitamins, and minerals that support optimal brain function. Nutrients such as omega-3 fatty acids (from chia seeds, flaxseeds, and walnuts), vitamin B12, magnesium, and folate play essential roles in mood regulation, nerve health, and energy production. By reducing processed foods and focusing on nutrient-dense plant sources, vegans may experience improved focus, emotional balance, and a sense of clarity.

Reduced Inflammation and Improved Mood

Research suggests that chronic inflammation can contribute to depression and anxiety. A vegan diet, naturally lower in saturated fats and higher in anti-inflammatory compounds like phytonutrients and flavonoids, helps reduce inflammation throughout the body and brain leading to more stable moods and emotional well-being.

The Gut–Mind Connection

Over 90% of serotonin the "feel-good" neurotransmitter is produced in the gut. A vegan diet, high in fiber from fruits, vegetables, legumes, and whole grains, supports a healthy gut microbiome. This promotes better digestion and stronger communication between the gut and brain, helping to enhance mood and reduce symptoms of stress, fatigue, and anxiety.

Emotional Alignment and Compassion

Veganism is not only a dietary choice—it's a lifestyle rooted in compassion, mindfulness, and intentional living. Many who adopt a vegan lifestyle report feeling more connected to their values, experiencing inner peace and emotional alignment by knowing their choices contribute to kindness toward all living beings. This emotional integrity often fosters self-respect, purpose, and a deeper sense of calm.

Mindful Living and Reduced Stress

Choosing veganism often encourages greater mindfulness—awareness of what we consume, how it affects us, and the world around us. This conscious living can extend beyond food, reducing emotional clutter and promoting gratitude, self-care, and spiritual well-being.

Veganism and Mental Health: Nourishing the Mind, Body, and Spirit

The Science Behind Nutrition and Mental Wellness

Our brains rely on a steady supply of nutrients to function optimally. A balanced vegan diet provides an abundance of vitamins, minerals, and plant-based compounds that nurture brain health and mood balance.

Key nutrients and their mental health benefits include:
- Omega-3 fatty acids (from flaxseed, chia, hemp, walnuts, and algae oil) essential for brain cell integrity and emotional regulation.
- Vitamin B12 (via fortified foods or supplements) supports the nervous system and prevents fatigue and mood swings.
- Folate (found in dark leafy greens, lentils, and avocado) critical for serotonin production.
- Magnesium (in spinach, almonds, and pumpkin seeds) helps calm the nervous system and reduce anxiety.
- Antioxidants (from colorful fruits and vegetables) protect the brain from oxidative stress.

Studies show that individuals following plant-based diets experience lower levels of stress and anxiety compared to those consuming meat-heavy diets.

Reducing Inflammation, Increasing Joy

Chronic inflammation has been identified as a contributor to depression and anxiety. A plant-based diet, rich in anti-inflammatory foods like berries, leafy greens, turmeric, and legumes, helps protect against mood disturbances.

"When the body is at peace, the mind can follow." - Dr. Neal Barnard

The Gut–Brain Connection: Healing from the Inside Out

Over 90% of the body's serotonin the neurotransmitter responsible for happiness and well-being is produced in the gut. A vegan diet supports a diverse gut microbiome through fiber-rich foods, which help communicate directly with the brain and reduce anxiety.

Emotional Alignment and Compassionate Living

Choosing not to participate in harm fosters a sense of peace, empathy, and moral integrity. This deep alignment between heart and action can create profound emotional stability and inner calm.

"The greatest peace comes from knowing you are doing no harm." - Anonymous

Spiritual and Mindful Healing

Veganism naturally encourages mindfulness awareness of what we consume and how it affects the world. As individuals shift toward conscious eating, they often experience greater focus, creativity, emotional regulation, and spiritual clarity.

Managing Stress and Emotional Fatigue Naturally

Stress is a normal part of life, but nutrition can determine how our bodies respond to it. Foods rich in vitamin C, magnesium, and complex carbohydrates help regulate cortisol levels the body's primary stress hormone.

The Bigger Picture: Veganism as a Mental Health Movement

The impact of veganism extends beyond individual health it influences global consciousness. By choosing plant-based living, individuals become part of a movement that promotes sustainability, compassion, and collective peace.

In Essence

Veganism is a lifestyle of nourishment, compassion, and mindfulness a holistic path toward both physical and mental liberation. By choosing plants, we choose peace for our minds, our bodies, and the world.

In Summary

Veganism nourishes more than just the body it supports a balanced mind and a compassionate heart. By embracing plant-based living, individuals often experience improved mood, mental clarity, and a renewed sense of harmony between their physical health, emotional wellness, and moral values.

🍲 Practical Living: Bringing Veganism into Everyday Life

Veganism isn't just about removing animal products it's about *adding life, love, and awareness* to the way we eat and live.
This section is designed to help readers turn inspiration into action, giving them the tools, guidance, and confidence to live compassionately in the real world.

Living vegan is not complicated it's intentional. With a few mindful adjustments, your kitchen, shopping habits, and daily routines can align with your values and nourish your health at the same time.

🧺 Stocking a Vegan Pantry

Your pantry is the heart of your kitchen it's where health begins. A well-stocked vegan pantry ensures that nutritious, flavorful meals are always within reach.

🌽 Whole Grains

- Brown rice, quinoa, bulgur, barley, farro, millet, oats
- Great for building nourishing bowls, breakfast porridges, and grain salads.

🥫 Legumes

- Lentils (red, green, black), chickpeas, black beans, kidney beans
- Provide fiber, protein, and heart-healthy nutrients.

🌰 Nuts & Seeds

- Almonds, walnuts, chia seeds, flaxseeds, hemp seeds, sunflower seeds, cashews
- Use in smoothies, sauces, granolas, or as healthy snacks.

🌻 Plant-Based Milks

- Almond, oat, soy, coconut, cashew, or rice milk
- Fortified options often contain B12, calcium, and vitamin D.

🫒 Healthy Oils & Condiments

- Olive oil, coconut oil, sesame oil
- Tamari, soy sauce, apple cider vinegar, tahini, mustard, and nutritional yeast.

🥫 Canned & Shelf-Stable Essentials

- Diced tomatoes, tomato paste, coconut milk, vegetable broth, nut butters
- Perfect for soups, sauces, and quick meals.

🌿 Herbs & Spices

- Garlic, onion, basil, turmeric, paprika, cumin, thyme, rosemary, ginger, and cinnamon
- Herbs and spices are the key to turning simple ingredients into vibrant meals.

"A vegan kitchen is not empty it's full of color, creativity, and compassion."

🛒 Smart Vegan Shopping Tips

Transitioning to vegan living begins with mindful shopping. With a little preparation, grocery shopping becomes an act of love for your health, the planet, and every living being.

💚 Plan Ahead

- Create a weekly menu before heading to the store.
- Make a checklist of pantry staples and fresh produce.

🥦 Shop the Perimeter

Most whole foods fruits, vegetables, grains are found around the outer aisles of grocery stores.
Avoid processed or prepackaged foods whenever possible.

🌱 Read Labels Carefully

Look out for hidden animal-derived ingredients such as:

- Whey, casein, gelatin, honey, or lard.
  Choose certified vegan labels when possible.

💵 Budget-Friendly Tip

Buy grains, legumes, and nuts in bulk.
Freeze fresh produce or cook in large batches to reduce waste and save money.

"Shopping with awareness turns every purchase into a statement of purpose."

Thriving On Plants

🌱 Everyday Cooking Made Simple

Cooking vegan meals doesn't require fancy skills just creativity and love. Once you learn a few basic techniques, you can prepare nourishing meals effortlessly.

🍲 Cooking Essentials

- **Batch cooking:** Prepare large portions of grains or beans to use throughout the week.
- **Flavor building:** Use sautéed onions, garlic, herbs, and spices to create depth.
- **Experimentation:** Try new vegetables, global spices, and sauces.

🍽 Quick Meal Ideas

- **Breakfast:** Smoothies, oatmeal with nuts and fruits, tofu scramble.
- **Lunch:** Veggie wraps, quinoa salad, or lentil soup.
- **Dinner:** Stir-fried veggies with rice, lentil curry, roasted chickpeas with greens.

💡 Cooking with Purpose

Cooking vegan is an act of creativity and care it connects you to your food and to the Earth.
When you prepare meals with love and gratitude, you feed not only your body but also your spirit.

"Cook with love, eat with joy, live with peace."

🏠 Transitioning Gracefully

For beginners, transitioning to veganism is a journey not a race. It's okay to start small and grow with time.

Thriving On Plants

🌱 Start Where You Are

- Begin by replacing one meal a day with a plant-based option.
- Explore vegan versions of your favorite dishes.

🍃 Progress Over Perfection

Don't be discouraged by mistakes or cravings. Every plant-based choice counts.
Forgive yourself for missteps and celebrate every small success.

🌼 Connect with Your Why

Remind yourself of the reason you began health, compassion, faith, or sustainability.
Keeping your purpose close will help you stay grounded on hard days.

"Every small choice rooted in love becomes a step toward transformation."

🧠 Nutrition & Balance

A balanced vegan diet is full of vitality when you eat a variety of foods.

🥦 Key Nutrients to Prioritize

- **Protein:** Beans, lentils, tofu, tempeh, quinoa, nuts, seeds.
- **Iron:** Spinach, lentils, chickpeas, pumpkin seeds, fortified cereals.
- **Calcium:** Fortified plant milks, tahini, almonds, kale, tofu.
- **Vitamin B12:** Supplement or fortified foods (very important).
- **Omega-3s:** Chia seeds, flaxseeds, hemp seeds, walnuts.

Thriving On Plants

😋 Mindful Eating

Sit, breathe, and bless your meal.
Be present while eating — enjoy textures, colors, and flavors.
This practice deepens your connection to food and your body's wisdom.

💰 Budget-Friendly Vegan Living

Veganism can be affordable with intentional planning.

🌽 Simple Tips

- Cook at home more often than dining out.
- Buy frozen fruits and vegetables they're nutritious and less expensive.
- Eat seasonally and locally.
- Avoid excessive processed vegan products.

"Healthy doesn't mean costly simplicity is the secret of nourishment."

👨🏿‍👩🏾‍👧🏽 Veganism for Families

Transitioning as a family can be joyful and bonding.

- Involve children in cooking and grocery shopping.
- Present meals creatively bright colors and fun textures encourage interest.
- Introduce plant-based versions of familiar dishes (vegan macaroni, tacos, or burgers).
- Share the *why* behind your choices in a loving, age-appropriate way.

"When families cook together, they grow together."

🥗 Dining Out & Social Gatherings

🍱 Eating Out

- Look for plant-based options at restaurants or use apps to locate vegan-friendly spots.
- Don't hesitate to ask for modifications most chefs are happy to help.

🎉 Social Events

- Bring a vegan dish to share it introduces others to delicious plant-based food.
- Focus on fellowship, not just food.
- Be kind and patient with loved ones who may not understand your choices.

"Kindness on your plate leads to kindness at every table."

🌍 Sustainable & Mindful Living

Veganism extends beyond food it's a holistic lifestyle of care for all creation.

🌱 Simple Acts of Eco-Compassion

- Use reusable bags, bottles, and containers.
- Choose cruelty-free cleaning and beauty products.
- Support ethical and fair-trade brands.
- Reduce waste by composting and recycling.

"Living vegan is living responsibly a love letter to the planet."

🌱 7-Day Vegan Starter Plan

Day 1: Smoothie + Lentil soup + Stir-fry
Day 2: Overnight oats + Buddha bowl + Veggie pasta
Day 3: Fruit salad + Chickpea wrap + Curry & rice
Day 4: Green juice + Quinoa salad + Roasted tofu & veggies
Day 5: Vegan pancakes + Hummus sandwich + Burrito bowl
Day 6: Avocado toast + Grain bowl + Spaghetti with vegan meatballs
Day 7: Fresh juice + Veggie burger + Coconut curry

"A week of vegan living can plant a lifetime of compassion."

Take your time for this new lifestyle. Change some days up and be creative. Make this your own and have fun while living plant-based.

Thriving On Plants

Thriving On Plants

PREPARE FOR THIS AMAZING JOURNEY…

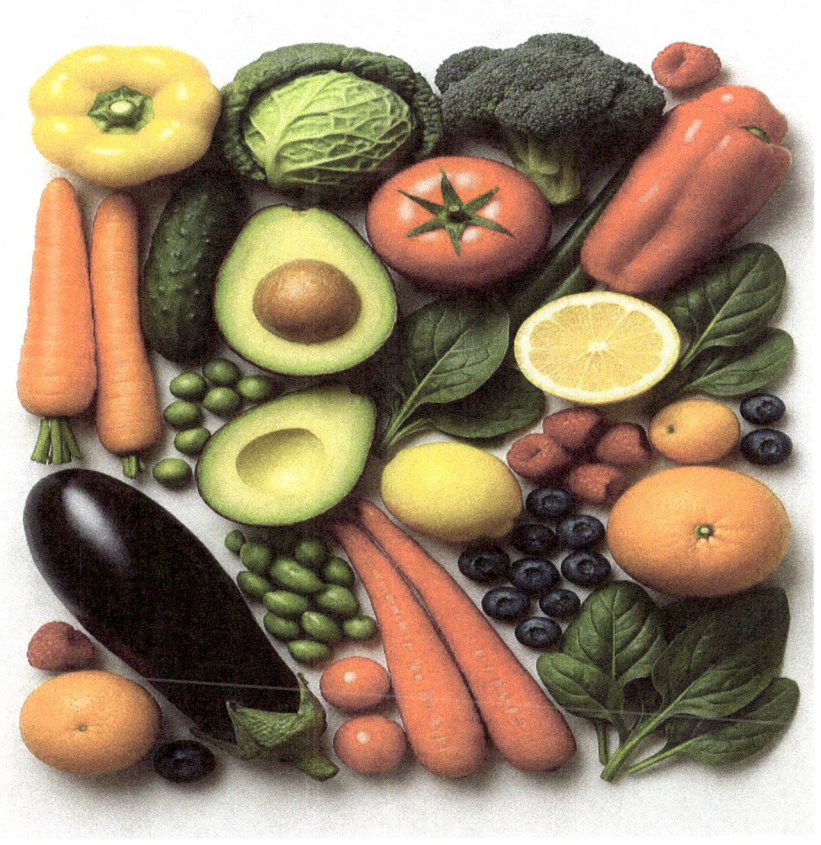

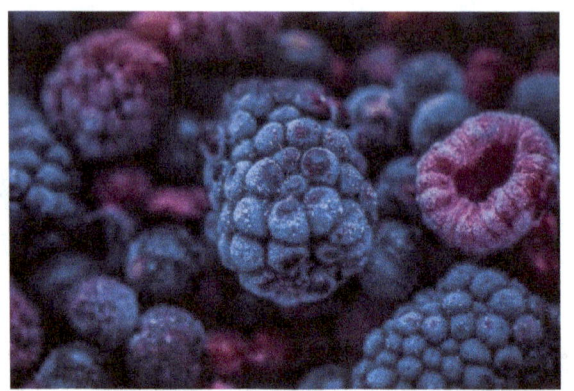

Chapter 1: Why Go Vegan for Health?

Thriving on Plants: A Health-First Guide to Going Vegan

Introduction:

A New Way of Eating for a New You

The food we eat shapes the way we feel, the way we age, and the way our bodies fight disease. For decades, the Western diet has revolved around heavy portions of meat, dairy, and processed foods. These foods are convenient and deeply ingrained in cultural traditions, but they've also been linked to rising rates of obesity, type 2 diabetes, cardiovascular disease, and certain cancers.

At the same time, research from leading nutrition scientists has uncovered a powerful truth: eating more plants can transform our health. Studies consistently show that people who eat a predominantly plant-based diet have lower risks of chronic illness, more energy, and even longer life expectancy.

For some, the motivation to go vegan stems from ethical or environmental concerns. For others, it comes from a place of necessity a wake-up call from a doctor, a family history of illness, or simply the desire to feel vibrant again. This book is written for those who want to embrace veganism **first and foremost for health reasons**.

Changing to a vegan lifestyle doesn't have to be overwhelming or restrictive. In fact, it can be liberating. You'll discover new flavors, new routines, and a renewed sense of well-being. By the end of this book, you'll understand not just the *why* but also the *how* to nourish yourself fully on plants, how to transition gracefully, and how to sustain this way of living long-term.

When people hear the word "vegan," they often think about animals or the environment. But for me, the journey began with something much closer to home: my health.

At the time, I was *feeling constantly tired, struggling with weight gain, and noticing my blood pressure creeping up*. I knew something had to change, but I wasn't sure what. I had tried *"low-carb diets, calorie counting, even skipping meals"*, and none of it seemed to stick.

One day, I started a 40 holistic diet that caused me to focus on eating to live, not living to eat. I stumbled across *an article about plant-based diets*. At first, the idea of giving up meat and dairy sounded extreme. But the more I learned about how a whole-food, plant-based diet could improve heart health, reduce inflammation, and give me steady energy, the more it clicked: this wasn't about restriction. This was about healing.

I decided to try it not as a lifelong commitment at first, but as an experiment. *What if I just gave it 30 days?*

The results surprised me. Within the first few weeks, I noticed *my digestion improved, I had more energy in the mornings, and I didn't feel that heavy afternoon crash anymore*. By the end of the month, I realized I didn't miss my old foods nearly as much as I thought I would. In fact, I felt lighter, both physically and mentally.

That's when it hit me: this wasn't just a diet. It was a new way of living one that supported my health rather than working against it.

And while every person's journey looks different, I discovered something important: food is one of the most powerful tools we have for changing our health. With every plant-based meal, I was taking control of my body, my future, and my story.

In this book, I want to share not only the science and strategies behind going vegan for health but also the lessons I learned along the way. Because if I could make this shift starting exactly where I was, I believe you can, too.

The Evidence for Plant-Based Eating

Let's start with the facts. Decades of medical research has built a strong case for plant-based eating:

- **Heart health:** Plant-based diets are naturally low in saturated fat and cholesterol, which are strongly linked to heart disease. A landmark study published in the *Journal of the American Heart Association* found that those who consumed the most plant-based foods had a **16% lower risk of cardiovascular disease** and a **32% lower risk of death from cardiovascular causes** compared to those who ate the least.

- **Diabetes prevention and management:** Type 2 diabetes is one of the fastest-growing health challenges worldwide. Research shows that those who eat mostly plant-based foods have a significantly reduced risk. A study from Harvard involving more than 200,000 participants found that a healthy plant-based diet lowered diabetes risk by 34%.

- **Cancer risk reduction:** The World Health Organization has classified processed meat as a carcinogen and red meat as a probable carcinogen. Meanwhile, diets rich in fruits, vegetables, legumes, and whole grains provide protective antioxidants, fiber, and phytochemicals that lower cancer risk.

- **Longevity and vitality:** The "Blue Zones" regions around the world where people live the longest, healthiest lives all share one common factor: their diets are overwhelmingly plant-based. From Okinawa, Japan to Loma Linda, California, plant foods dominate the plates of the world's longest-lived people.

Beyond Disease Prevention: Everyday Benefits

While the long-term protection against disease is compelling, the benefits of going vegan are felt almost immediately:

- **More energy:** Without the heaviness of animal fats and processed meats, many people report feeling lighter, more energized, and mentally clearer within weeks.
- **Improved digestion:** Plant-based diets are high in fiber, which supports gut health, regularity, and even mental well-being through the gut-brain connection.
- **Weight management:** Because plant foods tend to be lower in calories yet higher in nutrients and fiber, they naturally help with satiety and sustainable weight loss.
- **Glowing skin:** Antioxidants and vitamins from fruits and vegetables can reduce inflammation and support clearer, healthier skin.

Debunking the Myths

If plant-based diets are so healthy, why do so many people hesitate? Largely because of myths:

- **Myth 1: You won't get enough protein.**
  In reality, beans, lentils, tofu, tempeh, quinoa, seitan, nuts, and seeds provide plenty of protein. Most people easily meet their protein needs without animal products.
- **Myth 2: Vegan diets are restrictive.**
  Veganism opens the door to a vast variety of foods. There are thousands of edible plants, grains, legumes, and spices that most meat-centered diets ignore.
- **Myth 3: It's too difficult or expensive.**
  With some planning, vegan eating can be simple and

affordable. Staples like rice, beans, oats, and seasonal vegetables are among the cheapest foods in the grocery store.

- **Myth 4: You'll feel weak without meat.**
  Many elite athletes thrive on vegan diets, proving that plant foods provide all the strength, stamina, and recovery nutrients the human body needs.

Why Health-Focused Veganism Matters

Going vegan for health reasons doesn't mean you have to give up your cultural identity, your enjoyment of food, or your social life. It means making deliberate choices that prioritize your body's well-being. Unlike fad diets, this isn't about restriction, quick fixes, or chasing a number on the scale. It's about adopting a way of eating that is abundant, nourishing, and sustainable.

When you decide to change to a vegan lifestyle for health, you are:

- Taking control of your future well-being.
- Reducing your risk of preventable disease.
- Gaining energy and vitality for everyday life.
- Investing in a long, healthy life for yourself and your loved ones.

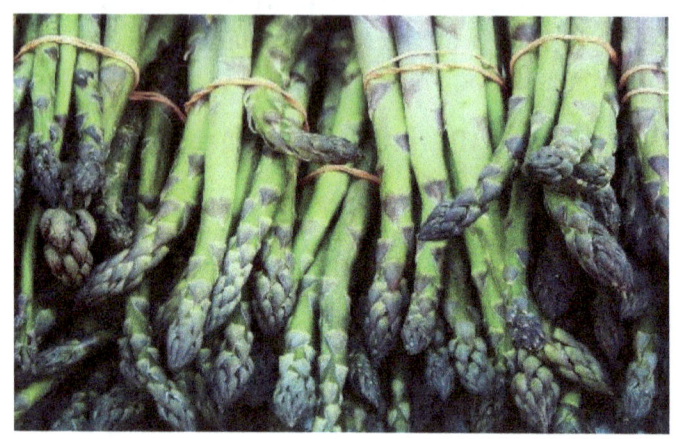

Chapter 2: Understanding Nutrition, the Vegan Way

When people first consider a vegan lifestyle, one of the most common worries is: *"Will I get all the nutrients I need?"* It's a fair question. After all, many of us grew up being told that milk was essential for strong bones, that meat was the only "real" source of protein, and that a balanced diet must include animal products.

The truth is that the human body is incredibly adaptable and capable of thriving on a diet made entirely of plants as long as you understand the basics of nutrition and make mindful choices.

This chapter will walk you through the essentials: macronutrients, micronutrients, and a few key nutrients to pay closer attention to on a vegan diet.

Macronutrients: Building Blocks of Energy and Strength

Macronutrients protein, fat, and carbohydrates are the foundation of every diet. Let's break down how they work in a vegan lifestyle.

Protein: The Muscle Builder

Protein is made up of amino acids, the "building blocks" of your body's tissues. Many people associate protein only with meat, but plants provide abundant sources.

Key vegan protein sources include:

- Legumes: lentils, chickpeas, black beans, kidney beans
- Soy products: tofu, tempeh, edamame
- Whole grains: quinoa, brown rice, oats, buckwheat
- Nuts and seeds: almonds, walnuts, chia seeds, hemp seeds, pumpkin seeds
- Seitan (wheat gluten): an especially protein-rich food, loved in vegan cooking

How much do you need?
Most adults require about **0.8–1 gram of protein per kilogram of**

body weight daily. For example, a 150-pound (68 kg) person needs around 55–68 grams of protein per day easily achievable with a varied vegan diet.

Fats: The Brain and Hormone Supporters

Fats are vital for brain function, hormone regulation, and nutrient absorption. While animal fats are high in cholesterol and saturated fat, plant fats tend to be rich in healthy unsaturated fats.

Key vegan fat sources include:

- Avocados
- Nuts (cashews, almonds, walnuts, pecans)
- Seeds (chia, flax, hemp, sunflower, sesame)
- Olives and olive oil
- Coconut (in moderation)

One important type of fat to pay attention to is **omega-3 fatty acids**, which support heart and brain health. Since fish is off the menu, the best vegan sources are flaxseeds, chia seeds, hemp seeds, walnuts, and algae-based supplements.

Carbohydrates: The Energy Fuel

Carbs have been unfairly demonized in modern diet culture, but they are the body's **preferred source of energy**. The key is choosing complex, fiber-rich carbohydrates rather than refined, sugary ones.

Healthy vegan carb sources include:

- Whole grains: brown rice, quinoa, oats, barley, millet
- Starchy vegetables: sweet potatoes, squash, corn
- Legumes: beans, lentils, peas
- Fruits: bananas, apples, berries, oranges

These foods provide long-lasting energy, fiber for digestion, and a wide range of vitamins and minerals.

Micronutrients: The Small but Mighty Essentials

Micronutrients vitamins and minerals are needed in smaller amounts than macronutrients, but they're absolutely critical for good health. Most are abundant in plant foods, but there are a few that require special attention on a vegan diet.

Vitamin B12

- **Why it matters:** Vital for red blood cell production and nervous system health.
- **Challenge:** B12 is not reliably available from plants because it's produced by bacteria (not animals themselves). In the modern food supply, it's found in animal products due to supplementation in animal feed.
- **Solution:** Every vegan should take a B12 supplement (or consume fortified foods like plant milks and nutritional yeast).

Iron

- **Why it matters:** Essential for oxygen transport in the blood.
- **Sources:** Lentils, chickpeas, black beans, tofu, spinach, pumpkin seeds, quinoa.
- **Tip:** Plant-based (non-heme) iron is absorbed more efficiently when paired with vitamin C. For example, squeeze lemon juice over spinach, or enjoy beans with tomatoes or bell peppers.

Calcium

- **Why it matters:** Supports bone strength and muscle function.
- **Sources:** Fortified plant milks, tofu made with calcium sulfate, kale, bok choy, almonds, tahini, broccoli.

- **Note:** You don't need dairy to build strong bones — plant sources are highly effective when consumed regularly.

Vitamin D

- **Why it matters:** Works with calcium to maintain strong bones and regulate immunity.
- **Sources:** Sunshine is the most natural source. In winter or in low-sun regions, a vitamin D supplement (preferably D2 or vegan D3 from lichen) may be helpful.

Zinc

- **Why it matters:** Supports immune function, wound healing, and cell growth.
- **Sources:** Pumpkin seeds, hemp seeds, cashews, chickpeas, lentils, oats, quinoa.

Iodine

- **Why it matters:** Essential for thyroid health.
- **Sources:** Sea vegetables (nori, kelp, wakame), iodized salt.

The Whole Foods, Plant-Based Advantage

The beauty of vegan nutrition lies in its abundance. Unlike restrictive diets that cut out entire food groups, a whole-foods vegan diet emphasizes variety: grains, beans, fruits, vegetables, nuts, and seeds. When you eat a colorful, balanced plate, you naturally get the nutrients you need and you avoid many of the harmful compounds found in animal products (like cholesterol and excess saturated fat).

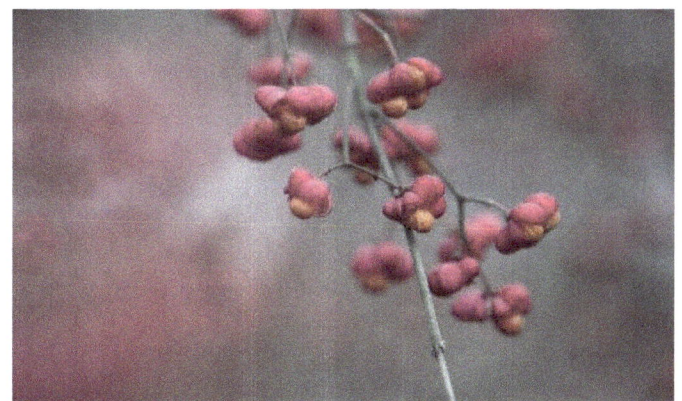

Chapter 3: Preparing for the Transition

Making the decision to go vegan for health reasons is exciting but like any lifestyle change, it's most successful when approached with preparation and intention. Going "cold turkey" works for some, but most people benefit from a gradual shift that allows their taste buds, routines, and mindset to adjust.

This chapter will guide you through the preparation process: assessing your current diet, setting health goals, and reframing the way you think about food.

Step 1: Assess Where You Are Now

Before making changes, it helps to get a clear picture of your current eating habits.

Keep a 3-Day Food Journal

For three typical days, write down everything you eat and drink — from your morning coffee to your evening snack. Be honest and don't change your habits for the journal. This record will help you:

- See how often you're eating animal products
- Notice patterns of processed foods or sugar
- Identify meals or snacks that could easily be "veganized"

For example, if you notice that breakfast often includes scrambled eggs, you can start thinking about plant-based alternatives like tofu scramble or overnight oats.

Look at Your Energy and Health Markers

Ask yourself:

- How is my energy throughout the day?
- Do I feel bloated, sluggish, or heavy after meals?
- Am I experiencing any health issues (e.g., high cholesterol, blood pressure, or digestive problems)?

These reflections give you a personal "baseline" so you can track improvements as you transition.

Step 2: Define Your Health Goals

Clarity is motivating. Knowing why you're making this change will keep you grounded when challenges arise.

Here are some common health-related goals people set when moving toward veganism:

- **Lowering cholesterol or blood pressure**
- **Improving digestion and gut health**
- **Losing weight in a sustainable way**
- **Increasing energy and mental clarity**
- **Reducing inflammation and joint pain**
- **Preventing or managing chronic disease**

Choose 1–3 goals that resonate most with you. Write them down somewhere visible on a sticky note by your fridge, in your journal, or as a note in your phone. These reminders will help when motivation dips.

Step 3: Shift Your Mindset

The transition to veganism isn't just about food; it's about perspective.

Think Addition, Not Restriction

Instead of focusing on what you're "giving up," focus on what you're adding:

- New flavors and cuisines
- Colorful produce you may have overlooked
- More energy and lighter digestion

- The joy of discovering foods that truly nourish your body

This mindset makes the journey feel expansive rather than limiting.

Release the All-or-Nothing Mentality

Perfection isn't the goal progress is. If you accidentally eat something with dairy or slip back into old habits, don't see it as failure. Instead, view it as feedback: what triggered the choice, and how can you prepare differently next time?

Remember, every plant-based meal is a win for your health.

Visualize Your Future Self

Picture yourself six months from now:

- How do you feel waking up in the morning?
- What does your energy look like throughout the day?
- How has your health improved?

This visualization helps anchor your motivation in a tangible outcome.

Step 4: Plan Your Transition Strategy

There's no one "right" way to go vegan. The best approach is the one that feels sustainable for you. Here are three common strategies:

1. Gradual Reduction

- Start by cutting out one category of animal products at a time.
  - Example: First cut out red meat, then poultry, then fish, then dairy, then eggs.
- Alternatively, start with one vegan meal per day (like breakfast) and build from there.

This works well for people who want a smooth transition without overwhelming their routines.

2. The 30-Day Challenge

- Commit to eating fully vegan for 30 days.
- Treat it like an experiment at the end, reflect on how you feel physically and emotionally.

This method provides a structured, time-bound challenge that many find motivating.

3. All-In, Right Now

- Remove all animal products from your kitchen immediately.
- Learn on the go, making quick swaps as needed.

This bold approach works best for people who thrive on commitment and immersion.

Step 5: Prepare Your Environment

Your surroundings play a big role in your success.

Clean Out Your Kitchen

- Remove or donate animal products you no longer want to eat.
- Replace them with plant-based staples (more on this in Chapter 4).

Stock Up on Quick Wins

Have easy, go-to meals ready for when hunger strikes:

- Cans of beans for quick chili or salads
- Pre-chopped veggies or frozen stir-fry mixes
- Plant-based milks for smoothies or cereal
- Nut butters and fruit for satisfying snacks

Gather Inspiration

Follow vegan recipe blogs, buy a beginner-friendly cookbook, or join online communities where people share meal ideas. Exposure to new recipes will keep your meals exciting and prevent boredom.

Step 6: Involve Your Support System

You don't have to do this alone. Share your health goals with family, friends, or even coworkers. You may inspire them to try new recipes with you, or at least they'll understand why you're making changes.

If you anticipate resistance, remember: this is *your* health journey. You don't need permission or approval to prioritize your well-being.

Takeaway: Preparation is the Foundation

Transitioning to a vegan lifestyle is less about willpower and more about preparation. By assessing your current habits, setting clear goals, shifting your mindset, and creating a supportive environment, you'll lay a strong foundation for success.

This isn't about being perfect it's about moving intentionally toward a healthier, plant-based life.

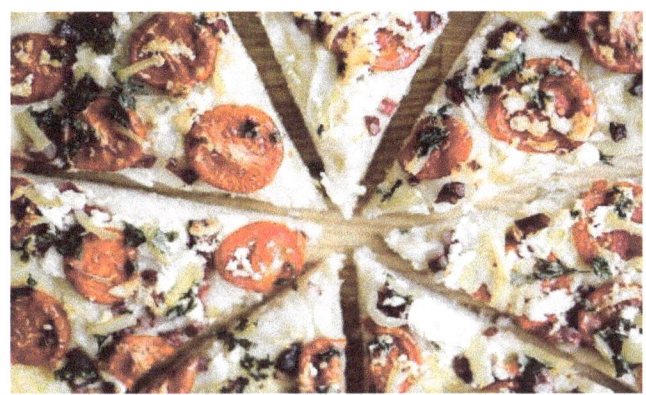

Chapter 4: Stocking Your Vegan Kitchen

Your kitchen is the foundation of your new lifestyle. If it's filled with nourishing plant-based foods, you'll find it easier and more enjoyable to make healthy choices. Think of this chapter as building your "vegan toolkit." With the right staples in your pantry, fridge, and freezer, you'll be able to whip up balanced meals without stress.

The Three Zones of a Vegan Kitchen

1. **Pantry** – Long-lasting dry goods that form the backbone of your meals.
2. **Fridge** – Fresh produce, condiments, and ready-to-use items.
3. **Freezer** – Frozen fruits, vegetables, and batch-cooked meals for busy days.

By keeping all three zones stocked, you'll always have healthy options within reach.

Pantry Essentials

The pantry is your best friend when it comes to quick, nourishing meals. These foods last a long time, are budget-friendly, and provide endless possibilities.

Grains

Grains provide energy, fiber, and essential minerals. Mix them up to keep your meals interesting.

- Brown rice
- Quinoa
- Oats (rolled or steel-cut)
- Barley
- Millet
- Buckwheat

- Whole-grain pasta

Legumes

Legumes are the cornerstone of plant-based protein. Keep both dried and canned versions on hand.

- Lentils (green, brown, red)
- Chickpeas
- Black beans
- Kidney beans
- Cannellini beans
- Split peas

Nuts and Seeds

These provide protein, healthy fats, and minerals.

- Almonds, cashews, walnuts, peanuts
- Sunflower seeds, pumpkin seeds, sesame seeds
- Chia, flax, and hemp seeds (great for omega-3s)
- Nut butters (peanut, almond, cashew, tahini)

Spices and Seasonings

Spices make healthy food exciting. Experiment and discover your favorites.

- Garlic powder, onion powder
- Cumin, coriander, turmeric
- Chili powder, smoked paprika
- Curry powder, garam masala

- Cinnamon, nutmeg, ginger
- Soy sauce, tamari, or coconut aminos
- Nutritional yeast (adds a cheesy, savory flavor and is fortified with B12)

Other Pantry Staples

- Canned tomatoes (diced, crushed, or pureed)
- Vegetable broth or bouillon cubes
- Whole-grain bread or wraps (store in the freezer if needed)
- Dried fruit (dates, raisins, cranberries)
- Dark chocolate (dairy-free for a healthy treat)

Fridge Staples

Your fridge should feel alive with fresh produce and versatile ingredients that keep meals vibrant and satisfying.

Vegetables

Aim for variety and color. Different pigments often mean different nutrients.

- Leafy greens: spinach, kale, arugula, romaine
- Cruciferous veggies: broccoli, cauliflower, Brussels sprouts, cabbage
- Root vegetables: carrots, beets, radishes
- Alliums: onions, garlic, leeks, scallions
- Peppers, cucumbers, zucchini, eggplant

Fruits

Fresh fruit is the perfect snack or breakfast topper.

- Apples, oranges, bananas, grapes
- Berries (strawberries, blueberries, raspberries)
- Citrus (lemons and limes for flavoring meals)
- Seasonal fruits like mango, pineapple, peaches, or pears

Plant-Based Proteins

- Tofu (firm for stir-fries, silken for smoothies or desserts)
- Tempeh (great for marinating and grilling)
- Seitan (high in protein, with a meaty texture)
- Edamame (protein-packed snack or salad topping)

Condiments and Flavor Boosters

- Mustard, hot sauce, salsa
- Hummus (or ingredients to make it fresh)
- Plant-based yogurt
- Dairy-free cheese (optional, for transition comfort foods)

Plant Milks

Stock a couple of different types for variety. Choose unsweetened versions when possible.

- Soy milk (highest in protein)
- Almond, oat, or cashew milk
- Coconut milk (best for curries and baking)

Freezer Staples

The freezer is your safety net. It helps you avoid takeout when life gets busy.

Frozen Vegetables

- Broccoli, peas, corn, spinach, mixed stir-fry blends
- These are flash-frozen at peak freshness and retain nutrients.

Frozen Fruits

- Berries, mango, pineapple, cherries, bananas (great for smoothies and oatmeal).

Batch-Cooked Meals

- Soups, stews, and curries portioned into containers for busy nights.
- Homemade veggie burgers or falafel patties.

Grains and Legumes

- Cooked rice, quinoa, or beans can be frozen in portions for quick meals.

Kitchen Tools That Make Life Easier

While you don't need fancy equipment, a few tools can make plant-based cooking faster and more enjoyable:

- **High-powered blender** – for smoothies, soups, sauces, and nut-based dressings.
- **Food processor** – for hummus, dips, veggie burgers, and chopping.
- **Sharp knives and cutting board** – make chopping veggies easier and safer.

- **Instant Pot or slow cooker** – great for cooking beans, grains, and soups with little effort.
- **Air fryer or good-quality oven tray** – for crispy roasted veggies and oil-free cooking.

Smart Swaps for Everyday Meals

Transitioning doesn't mean giving up your favorite dishes it means finding creative swaps:

- **Milk → plant milk** (almond, soy, oat)
- **Butter → olive oil, coconut oil, or vegan butter**
- **Cheese → nutritional yeast, cashew-based cheese, or dairy-free brands**
- **Ground beef → lentils, mushrooms, or seasoned tofu crumbles**
- **Eggs in baking → flaxseed or chia "egg"** (1 tbsp ground seeds + 3 tbsp water)
- **Mayonnaise → hummus, avocado, or vegan mayo**

Sample Vegan Pantry Meals

Here are a few quick ideas you can make with a well-stocked kitchen:

- **Chickpea Curry** – canned chickpeas + coconut milk + canned tomatoes + curry spices + spinach.
- **Lentil Soup** – lentils + carrots + onions + celery + veggie broth + spices.
- **Tofu Stir-Fry** – tofu + frozen mixed vegetables + soy sauce + garlic + brown rice.
- **Overnight Oats** – rolled oats + plant milk + chia seeds + frozen berries + nut butter.

- **Veggie Wrap** – whole-grain tortilla + hummus + fresh veggies + avocado.

Takeaway: Set Yourself Up for Success

When your kitchen is filled with wholesome plant-based ingredients, healthy eating becomes effortless. You won't need to rely on willpower — the choices you've made in advance will guide you toward vibrant, nutrient-rich meals every day. Remember, you don't have to buy everything at once. Start with a few staples, experiment, and gradually build a pantry and fridge that make you excited to cook.

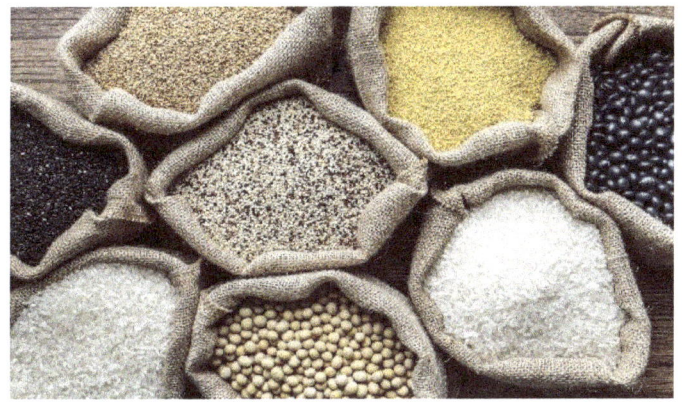

Chapter 5: The First 30 Days

The first month of your vegan journey is about building momentum, experimenting with new foods, and setting yourself up for long-term success. Think of this as your transition "training period." You're not aiming for perfection you're building habits, learning what works for your body, and proving to yourself that you can thrive on plants.

To make things simple, we'll divide the first month into **four weekly phases**. Each phase builds on the last, gradually increasing your comfort level with plant-based eating.

Week 1: Breaking Old Habits

That first week was the hardest. My fridge looked completely different no "milk, eggs, deli meat", and instead I had, "beans, tofu, kale, spinach, almond milk".

I remember my first grocery trip feeling overwhelming. I stood in the aisle reading labels, realizing how many foods had hidden animal products. But little by little, I figured it out.

Physically, I noticed changes right away. "My digestion felt smoother, I wasn't as bloated, and I slept better". Emotionally, I felt proud even if I was still clumsy in the kitchen.

Week 2: New Energy

By the second week, something shifted. The meals started to feel less foreign and more natural. I got into a rhythm with "oatmeal for breakfast, big salads for lunch, stir-fries for dinner".

I was surprised to notice my energy. Normally, I'd get an afternoon slump around 3 p.m. But now, I felt steady and alert. It was like my body was saying, *finally, thank you.*

Week 3: Social Challenges

Then came the real test: eating with others.

That week, I went out of town to a family dinner. I was nervous would I find something to eat? Would people judge me?

It wasn't perfect. I had to explain myself a couple of times, and I definitely got some curious looks. But I survived and more importantly, I realized that social situations were not deal-breakers. With a little planning, I could still enjoy time with others without compromising my new choices.

Week 4: Feeling the Difference

By the fourth week, veganism no longer felt like an "experiment." It was becoming my new normal.

Physically, I noticed clearer skin, less joint pain, or weight loss". Mentally, I felt sharper. And emotionally, I felt proud of sticking with it.

Most importantly, I realized I didn't want to go back. What started as a 30-day trial had become a lifestyle I actually enjoyed.

What I Learned in 30 Days

- The hardest part is starting after that, momentum carries you.
- Planning meals ahead of time makes everything easier.
- Energy doesn't come from willpower it comes from what you fuel your body with.
- Social situations are challenges, not roadblocks.
- Change happens faster than you think when you stay consistent.

Looking back, those first 30 days were about more than food. They were about proving to myself that I could change. If I could stick with it for a month through cravings, doubts, and social tests I could stick with it long term.

That's the power of the first 30 days. They don't just change your plate. They change your belief in what's possible.

Week 1: Starting Strong with Breakfasts and Snacks

Instead of overhauling your entire diet at once, begin with two easy categories: **breakfast and snacks**. These meals are often simpler, quicker, and less emotionally tied to tradition.

Action Steps

- Replace dairy milk with plant-based milk in cereal, coffee, or smoothies.
- Swap eggs with oatmeal, tofu scramble, or chia pudding.
- Keep fresh fruit, nuts, and hummus with veggies on hand for snacks.
- Experiment with 2–3 new vegan breakfast recipes this week.

Sample Breakfasts

- Overnight oats with almond milk, chia seeds, and berries
- Tofu scramble with spinach, mushrooms, and salsa
- Smoothie with banana, spinach, peanut butter, and soy milk
- Whole-grain toast with avocado and tomato

Snack Ideas

- Apple slices with almond butter
- Carrots and hummus
- Handful of walnuts and dried cranberries
- Rice cakes with peanut butter

Week 2: Transforming Lunches

Now that your mornings and snacks are plant-powered, it's time to tackle lunch. Lunches can be quick and portable, making them perfect for experimenting with hearty, satisfying vegan meals.

Action Steps

- Prep grain bowls, wraps, or hearty salads.
- Try replacing meat with beans, lentils, or tofu in your favorite dishes.
- Keep simple staples ready in the fridge (cooked rice, roasted veggies, beans).

Sample Lunches

- Quinoa bowl with roasted sweet potato, black beans, kale, and tahini dressing
- Chickpea salad sandwich (mashed chickpeas, vegan mayo, celery, lemon, herbs)
- Lentil soup with whole-grain bread
- Hummus and veggie wrap with spinach, cucumbers, and shredded carrots

Tip for Success

Batch cook 1–2 big items (like a pot of lentils or a tray of roasted vegetables) each week. Mix and match them with different sauces and grains for quick lunches.

Week 3: Reinventing Dinner

Dinners are often the hardest meal to change, since they're tied to tradition, family routines, and comfort. But by now, you'll already have breakfast, snacks, and lunch covered so dinner is the final piece of the puzzle.

Action Steps

- Choose 3–4 go-to vegan dinners you enjoy and rotate them.
- Use "smart swaps" for your old favorites (lentil tacos instead of beef tacos, chickpea curry instead of chicken curry).

- Cook double portions and save leftovers for the next day.

Sample Dinners

- Lentil chili with brown rice
- Stir-fried tofu with mixed vegetables and soba noodles
- Vegan curry with chickpeas, coconut milk, and spinach
- Baked sweet potato topped with black beans, salsa, and avocado
- Veggie burgers with roasted potato wedges

Tip for Success

Flavor is everything. Don't hold back on spices, herbs, or sauces. A bland meal will make you miss old habits, but a flavorful dish will leave you satisfied.

Week 4: Fine-Tuning and Full Commitment

By week four, you'll have experimented with a wide range of plant-based meals. Now it's time to reflect, refine, and commit.

Action Steps

- Review how you feel: energy levels, digestion, skin, mood.
- Identify your favorite recipes and make them your staples.
- Begin exploring restaurants or vegan-friendly options when dining out.
- Commit to trying at least one new recipe or ingredient per week going forward.

Experiment Ideas

- Try a new cuisine (Ethiopian lentils, Thai curry, Mediterranean mezze).

- Explore a new ingredient (tempeh, jackfruit, seitan).
- Bake something vegan (banana bread, muffins, cookies with flax "eggs").

Tip for Success

Don't get stuck in a rut of eating the same few meals. Variety is key to getting all your nutrients and keeping things exciting.

Handling Cravings in the First 30 Days

Cravings are normal when making any big dietary change. The key is to understand what your body and mind are really asking for.

- **Craving meat?** Try hearty, umami-rich foods like mushrooms, lentil stews, seitan, or soy sauce-flavored dishes.
- **Craving cheese?** Nutritional yeast, cashew-based cheeses, or hummus can satisfy that creamy, savory desire.
- **Craving sweets?** Choose fresh fruit, dark chocolate, or dates stuffed with peanut butter.
- **Craving comfort food?** Veganize your favorite dish mac and cheese, pizza, burgers with plant-based swaps.

Remember, cravings don't mean you're failing. They're simply signals that your body is adjusting.

Celebrating Wins and Progress

At the end of your first 30 days, take stock of your journey:

- How has your energy changed?
- How do your digestion and skin feel?
- Have you noticed shifts in mood or sleep?
- What health markers (like blood pressure or weight) have improved?

Even small improvements are worth celebrating. The first month is just the beginning but it's the most important step in creating a new normal.

Takeaway: Build Habits, Not Perfection

The first 30 days are about momentum, not mastery. By gradually transitioning through breakfasts, snacks, lunches, and dinners, you'll make the process manageable and enjoyable. Along the way, cravings will fade, energy will increase, and your confidence in plant-based eating will grow.

When you look back, you'll realize: *this isn't a diet, it's a lifestyle.*

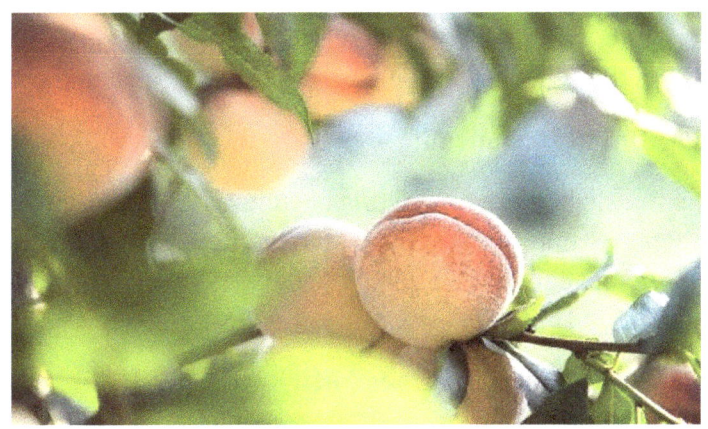

Chapter 6: Eating Out & Social Life

Changing what you eat at home is one thing but navigating restaurants, family gatherings, holidays, and travel can feel like a whole new challenge. The good news? With a little preparation and confidence, you can thrive socially and still honor your health goals.

This chapter will give you a **survival guide** for staying vegan without stress, including restaurant strategies, social scripts, and travel hacks.

Eating Out at Restaurants

Restaurants can feel intimidating at first, especially if your friends or family prefer traditional spots with meat-heavy menus. But with some creativity and communication, you can almost always find something satisfying.

Step 1: Scout the Menu Ahead of Time

- Most restaurants post their menus online. A quick look before you go helps you plan in advance.
- Look for keywords like: *vegetarian, grilled veggies, rice bowls, hummus, lentils, beans, salads, tofu.*

Step 2: Call Ahead (Optional but Powerful)

A quick phone call with:

"Hi, I'm vegan for health reasons. Could you prepare something without meat, dairy, or eggs?"
Most chefs enjoy the challenge and will often surprise you with something creative.

Step 3: Master the Art of Modification

You don't need a special vegan menu you just need confidence to ask for swaps.

- "Could I have the veggie burger without cheese or mayo?"
- "Can I get the stir-fry with tofu instead of chicken?"

- "I'd love the salad could you swap the dressing for olive oil and lemon?"

Step 4: Know Your Go-To Cuisines

Some cuisines are naturally vegan-friendly:

- **Mediterranean:** hummus, falafel, tabbouleh, roasted vegetables, pita
- **Indian:** chana masala (chickpeas), dal (lentils), aloo gobi (potatoes and cauliflower)
- **Thai:** veggie curries with coconut milk, tofu stir-fries, rice noodles
- **Ethiopian:** lentil stews, injera bread, veggie platters
- **Mexican:** bean burritos, veggie tacos, rice and guacamole

Navigating Social Gatherings

Food is often at the center of social life holidays, birthdays, family dinners. At first, you may worry about standing out, but there are plenty of ways to handle these situations gracefully.

Strategy 1: Offer to Bring a Dish

This is the simplest, most effective approach. Not only does it guarantee you'll have something to eat, but it also gives others a chance to taste how delicious vegan food can be.

Examples:

- Lentil chili
- Vegan lasagna with cashew cheese
- Roasted veggie platter with hummus
- Quinoa salad with herbs and lemon

Strategy 2: Communicate Ahead of Time

"I've been eating plant-based for health, so I'll bring a dish to share. That way I'll have something too and hopefully everyone can try it!"

This avoids putting pressure on your host while keeping you comfortable.

Strategy 3: Focus on the Social, Not Just the Food

Remember, gatherings are about connection, not just meals. If food options are limited, snack beforehand and focus on conversation.

Dealing with Questions (and Critics)

When you change your diet, some people will be curious and others might be skeptical. How you respond sets the tone.

Common Questions & Friendly Responses

- *"Where do you get your protein?"*
  "From beans, lentils, tofu, nuts there are so many great sources!"

- *"Don't you miss meat?"*
  "Honestly, I've found new foods I love. And I feel so much better."

- *"That sounds hard."*
  "It's easier than I thought once I learned a few new recipes."

Keep answers light and positive. You're not obligated to defend your choices your health is personal.

Traveling Vegan

Traveling adds another layer of challenge, but with planning, it can be exciting instead of stressful.

Before You Go

- Use apps like **Happy Cow** to find vegan-friendly restaurants worldwide.
- Pack snacks: nuts, trail mix, protein bars, dried fruit, instant oats.

On the Road

- Airports often have fruit, salads, or grain bowls.
- Gas stations usually have bananas, pretzels, or nut mixes.

At Your Destination

- Book accommodations with a kitchen if possible (Airbnb, extended stay hotels).
- Visit local markets fresh produce and regional plant foods are often the highlight of travel.
- Don't be afraid to ask locals for vegan-friendly dishes many traditional cuisines are naturally plant-based.

Mindset for Social Success

The key to navigating social life as a vegan is **confidence, flexibility, and preparation**.

- **Confidence:** Own your choices without apology. You're doing this for your health.
- **Flexibility:** Focus on what you *can* eat, not what you can't.
- **Preparation:** Always have a backup plan (snacks, a dish to share, or a restaurant option in mind).

Remember: every situation gets easier with practice. The first few dinners out may feel awkward, but soon it will become second nature.

Takeaway: Thrive Anywhere, Anytime

Being vegan isn't about isolating yourself it's about learning how to thrive in any environment. With a little creativity, you'll discover that restaurants, gatherings, and travel can be full of plant-based joy.

Instead of feeling left out, you'll feel empowered because no matter where you are, you'll know how to nourish your body and stick to your health goals.

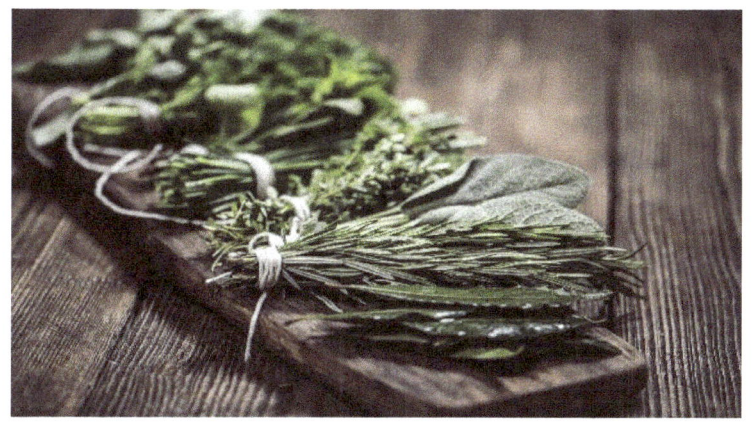

Chapter 7: Fitness and Energy on Plants

One of the most persistent myths about veganism is that it makes you weak, tired, or incapable of building muscle. In reality, a well-planned plant-based diet can fuel every level of fitness from weekend joggers to Olympic athletes. In fact, many people find their energy improves once they cut out heavy animal-based foods.

This chapter will explore how to maintain strength, stamina, and vitality on plants. You'll learn how to build muscle, recover effectively, and fuel your workouts with plant-based nutrition.

Energy from Plants: How It Works

At the most basic level, energy comes from calories the fuel your body burns to power everything from breathing to sprinting. The quality of those calories, however, makes all the difference.

- **Carbohydrates = Quick and Clean Energy**
  Whole plant foods like oats, rice, beans, and fruit provide steady, slow-burning fuel thanks to their fiber content. Unlike refined carbs, they prevent energy crashes.

- **Protein = Repair and Growth**
  After exercise, protein helps repair muscle tissue. Plant sources like beans, tofu, tempeh, seitan, quinoa, and nuts provide all the amino acids you need.

- **Fats = Endurance and Brain Power**
  Healthy fats from avocados, nuts, seeds, and olives keep you satiated and support long-term energy during endurance activities.

When these macronutrients come from whole plant sources, they deliver not just energy, but also fiber, antioxidants, and micronutrients that speed recovery and reduce inflammation.

Building Muscle on Plants

Muscle growth comes down to two key factors: **progressive resistance training** and **adequate protein intake**. A vegan diet can support both.

How Much Protein Do You Need?

- For general health: **0.8–1 g per kg of body weight**
- For active people: **1.2–2 g per kg of body weight**

That means a 150 lb (68 kg) person aiming to build muscle should aim for 80–120 grams of protein daily. This is easily achievable with beans, lentils, tofu, tempeh, seitan, soy milk, quinoa, and protein-rich snacks like nuts or smoothies.

Sample High-Protein Vegan Foods

- 1 cup lentils = 18 g
- 1 block firm tofu = 35 g
- 1 cup cooked quinoa = 8 g
- 2 tbsp peanut butter = 8 g
- 1 scoop vegan protein powder = 20–25 g

Example: Post-Workout Recovery Smoothie

- 1 scoop vegan protein powder (pea, hemp, or soy-based)
- 1 banana (quick carbs for glycogen refill)
- 1 cup spinach (micronutrients)
- 1 tbsp peanut butter (healthy fat)
- 1 cup soy milk (protein + calcium)

Total: ~30 g protein + carbs + fat for a balanced recovery.

Endurance and Stamina

Plant-based diets are naturally high in carbohydrates, which makes them ideal for endurance athletes like runners, cyclists, and swimmers. Carbs are stored as **glycogen** in the muscles and liver, providing the primary energy source for long workouts.

Many endurance athletes who go vegan report:

- Faster recovery times
- Less inflammation and soreness
- Improved digestion and lighter feeling during training

Pre-Workout Fuel

- Banana + handful of dates
- Oatmeal with berries and chia seeds
- Whole-grain toast with almond butter

During Long Workouts (90+ minutes)

- Energy gels or dried fruit
- Homemade date-and-oat energy balls
- Coconut water for electrolytes

Post-Workout

- Carbs to replenish glycogen + protein for muscle repair (rice and beans, lentil stew, smoothie).

Reducing Inflammation and Speeding Recovery

One of the biggest hidden advantages of a vegan diet for fitness is **anti-inflammatory power**.

Animal products are high in saturated fat and compounds that can promote inflammation. Plant foods, on the other hand, are packed with antioxidants, polyphenols, and omega-3 fatty acids that reduce inflammation.

This means:

- Less soreness after workouts
- Faster healing between sessions
- Reduced risk of chronic injury

Foods that are particularly powerful for recovery:

- Berries (antioxidants)
- Leafy greens (iron, calcium, magnesium)
- Turmeric + black pepper (anti-inflammatory)
- Chia and flax seeds (omega-3s)

Real-World Plant-Based Athletes

You don't have to take my word for it some of the strongest and fastest people in the world thrive on plants.

- **Patrik Baboumian** (World record–holding strongman): "I'm stronger than ever since going vegan. Who says you need meat to be strong?"
- **Venus Williams** (Tennis champion): Adopted a raw vegan diet to manage an autoimmune condition and returned to elite competition.
- **Scott Jurek** (Ultramarathon runner): Won multiple 100+ mile races on a plant-based diet.
- **Dotsie Bausch** (Olympic cyclist): Credits her vegan diet for improved recovery and performance at the highest level.

These athletes prove that strength, endurance, and recovery can all be maximized on plants.

Everyday Fitness and Energy

You don't have to be a professional athlete to reap the benefits. Whether your goal is keeping up with your kids, hiking on weekends, or just feeling good at the gym, plant foods provide sustainable energy.

Many people report:

- No more post-lunch "crashes"
- More consistent energy throughout the day
- Improved sleep and recovery at night

Takeaway: Powered by Plants

Fitness and veganism go hand in hand. By fueling your body with nutrient-dense carbs, plant proteins, and anti-inflammatory foods, you'll not only support your workouts but also feel more energized in daily life.

Going vegan for health isn't about losing strength it's about unlocking *more* of your body's potential.

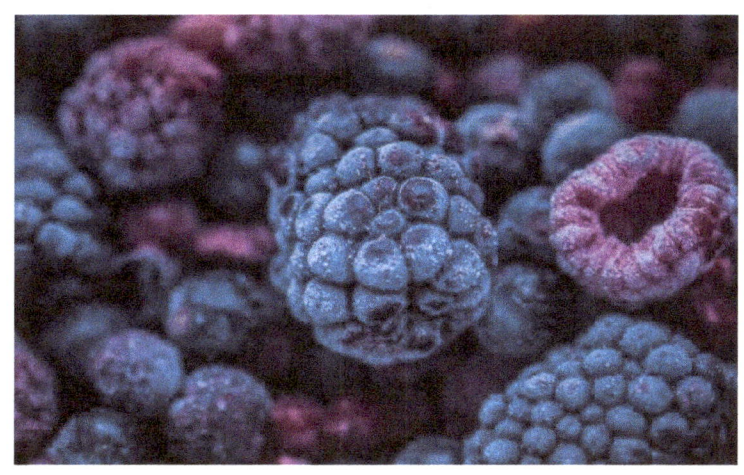

Chapter 8: Common Challenges and How to Overcome Them

No matter how motivated you are, every lifestyle change comes with hurdles. The path to health isn't always a straight line it's filled with cravings, slip-ups, awkward social moments, and unexpected learning curves.

In this chapter, we'll explore real-world struggles many new vegans face. Each story will highlight a challenge, the feelings that come with it, and the strategies that turned things around.

No matter how motivated you are, every lifestyle change comes with hurdles. Going vegan for health is no different. But here's the truth: challenges aren't signs of failure they're part of the process. Each one is a chance to grow stronger in your commitment.

When I started, I quickly realized that my journey wasn't just about learning new recipes. It was about unlearning old habits, handling social pressures, and finding confidence in my choices. Here are the challenges I faced and how I overcame them.

1. Cravings and Comfort Foods

In the beginning, I really missed eating cheesy foods, desserts, turkey hot dogs and pasta. It wasn't just the taste it was the memories and routines tied to those foods. Friday nights didn't feel the same without drinking wine and eating my favorite comfort foods (pasta, and desserts).

What helped me was finding plant-based swaps that satisfied those cravings. I discovered plant-based desserts. Were they identical? Not at first. But my taste buds adjusted, and soon they became my new comfort foods.

Lesson: You don't have to give up comfort just reinvent it.

2. Eating Out

One of my first social hurdles was going out to eat at my favorite restaurant for my birthday". The menu was stacked against me, and I worried I'd either go hungry or feel awkward.

What I learned was simple: plan ahead. Now I always look at menus online, call ahead, or suggest restaurants I know have vegan options". And more often than not, I find something delicious.

Lesson: With a little preparation, restaurants become less stressful and more enjoyable.

3. Family and Friends

Perhaps the hardest challenge was explaining my new lifestyle to the people I love. At first, my family's/friends' reaction, "they teased me, told me I'd never get enough protein, or kept offering me old favorites".

It wasn't easy, but I found that leading by example worked better than debating. Over time, they noticed my energy and health improvements. Some even got curious enough to try my recipes.

Lesson: Change invites resistance at first but consistency inspires respect.

4. Convenience and Busy Days

There were days I didn't want to cook. Days I felt too tired, too busy, too tempted to just grab something quick. That's when I realized the importance of having **go-to meals** ready.

I started keeping "frozen veggie stir-fry, cans of beans, whole-grain wraps, and hummus" stocked. Even on my worst days, I could throw something together in minutes.

Lesson: Prep isn't about being fancy it's about making the healthy choice the easy choice.

5. Slip-Ups

I'll be honest, I slipped up. There was a moment when I ate a slice of cheese and crackers at a party, or gave in to ice cream. At first, I felt guilty, like I had ruined everything.

But then I reminded myself: one slip doesn't erase the progress I've made. The next meal was another chance to get back on track.

Lesson: Perfection isn't the goal. Progress is.

Moving Through Challenges

Looking back, each struggle taught me something valuable. Cravings showed me the power of new flavors. Social challenges taught me confidence. Slip-ups taught me resilience.

The truth is, challenges don't end after the first month they evolve. But so do you. With every hurdle, you get stronger, more resourceful, and more confident in your choices.

And before long, what once felt like a struggle becomes second nature.

Story 1: Digestive Surprises

When *Laura*, a 36-year-old teacher, went vegan, she expected to feel lighter and energized. Instead, during the first two weeks, she felt bloated and gassy. She panicked: *"Maybe this isn't for me. My stomach is worse than before!"*

But what Laura didn't realize was that her gut microbiome the trillions of bacteria in her digestive system was adjusting to a sudden increase in fiber. She had gone from barely 15 grams of fiber a day to over 35 grams overnight.

What helped:

- She gradually reduced processed foods while easing into beans and cruciferous veggies.
- She soaked beans before cooking and started with smaller portions.
- Within three weeks, her gut adapted, and digestion improved dramatically.

Laura now laughs about it: *"My stomach just needed training — kind of like the rest of me."*

Story 2: The Cheese Craving

Marcus, a 42-year-old software engineer, had no problem giving up meat, but cheese was another story. He loved pizza nights with his kids and missed the gooey, salty taste. "I could go without steak forever," he said, "but cheese… I dream about it."

This is a common challenge. Cheese contains casein, a dairy protein that releases casomorphins compounds that can trigger pleasure receptors in the brain, making it genuinely addictive.

What helped:

- Marcus experimented with cashew-based cheeses and nutritional yeast ("nooch") for that cheesy, nutty flavor.
- Instead of giving up pizza, he started making his own with homemade cashew mozzarella and plenty of veggies.
- The cravings eased as his taste buds adjusted, and now he says: *"It's not the same, but honestly, I like my version better."*

Story 3: Eating Out Awkwardness

Jasmine, a college student, dreaded going out with friends after going vegan. Her friends loved burgers, wings, and BBQ joints. She didn't want to seem "difficult," but also didn't want to compromise her health.

At first, she just ordered French fries or a side salad and went home hungry. One night, she nearly caved and ordered chicken wings just to avoid questions.

What helped:

- She started suggesting new restaurants with vegan options (Thai, Mexican, Mediterranean).

- When friends insisted on BBQ, she called ahead and asked if the kitchen could make a veggie plate and they did!
- She learned to confidently say: *"I eat plant-based for my health, I'll find something, no worries."*

Now, her friends sometimes try her meals, and Jasmine realizes she didn't have to choose between health and belonging.

Story 4: The Social Pressure

Daniel, a 55-year-old father, went vegan after his doctor warned him about high cholesterol. He felt amazing within a month, but his family wasn't thrilled. His wife worried about cooking "two meals," and his coworkers teased him at lunch. *"What's with the rabbit food?"* they joked.

Daniel admits: *"I almost gave up just to make things easier."*

What helped:

- He took on cooking for himself, showing his family how tasty his meals could be.
- He shared his doctor's report, showing how his cholesterol dropped 40 points.
- Over time, the teasing turned into curiosity. His coworkers now ask for his black bean chili recipe.

Daniel's story shows that sometimes, the hardest part isn't food it's the people around you. But persistence often inspires others.

Story 5: The Slip-Up

Sara, 28, was three months into her vegan journey when she grabbed a muffin at a coffee shop only to realize halfway through that it contained butter and eggs. She felt guilty, ashamed, and almost considered quitting altogether.

What helped:

- She reframed the slip-up: it wasn't failure, just a mistake.
- She reminded herself: *"This is about progress, not perfection."*
- She prepared by keeping vegan snacks in her bag to avoid "emergency" choices.

Now, she sees the muffin incident as part of her learning curve, not the end of the road.

The Common Thread

What ties these stories together? Each person faced challenges that could have derailed them. But by adjusting, experimenting, and staying flexible, they found solutions.

The lesson: Success in going vegan isn't about perfection — it's about persistence. Your cravings, digestion, and social circle may resist at first, but your health and confidence grow stronger each time you keep going.

Takeaway: Struggles are Stepping Stones

Every challenge is part of the journey. Instead of seeing struggles as signs of failure, treat them as teachers. Whether it's digestion, cravings, awkwardness, or slip-ups, there's always a way forward.

Remember: it's not about never stumbling it's about getting back up, again and again. That's what builds lasting change.

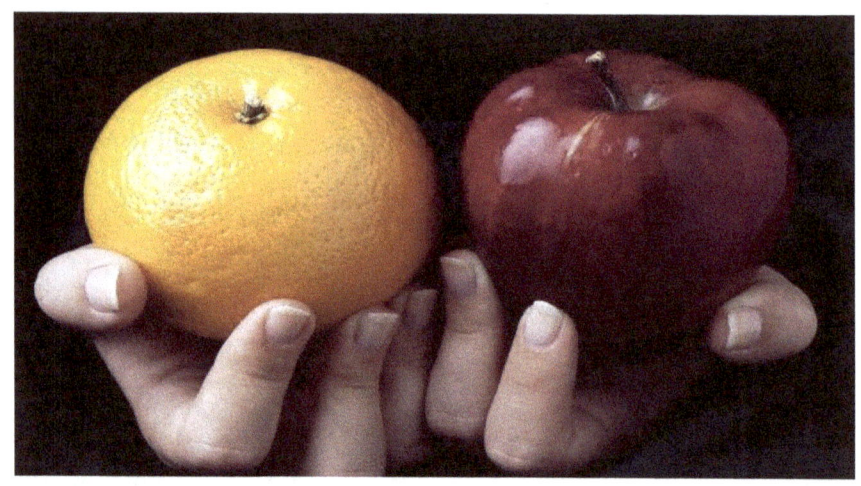

Chapter 9: Long-Term Sustainability

The first 30 days are exciting full of new flavors, fresh energy, and visible improvements in health. But what happens after the honeymoon phase? Sustainability is the true measure of success.

Going vegan for health isn't about a short-term cleanse; it's about building a lifestyle that supports you for years to come. The key lies in **structure**: creating routines, habits, and systems that make eating plant-based second nature.

1. Establishing Your Daily Routine

Consistency makes life easier. By creating a framework for your meals, you take the guesswork out of eating.

The Balanced Plate Method

For every main meal, aim for:

- **½ plate:** Vegetables and fruits (fiber, vitamins, antioxidants)
- **¼ plate:** Whole grains (brown rice, quinoa, oats, whole-wheat pasta)
- **¼ plate:** Plant protein (beans, lentils, tofu, tempeh, seitan)
- **1–2 tbsp:** Healthy fats (avocado, olive oil, nuts, seeds)

Daily Eating Flow Example

- **Breakfast:** Overnight oats with chia, soy milk, and berries
- **Snack:** Apple + peanut butter
- **Lunch:** Quinoa bowl with chickpeas, roasted broccoli, and tahini
- **Snack:** Carrots + hummus or a handful of almonds
- **Dinner:** Lentil curry with brown rice and spinach

2. Weekly Meal Planning

Planning ahead prevents stress and reduces the chance of "falling off" when life gets busy.

Step 1: Choose 3–4 Go-To Dinners

Rotate them weekly. Examples:

- Lentil chili
- Stir-fry with tofu and vegetables
- Vegan tacos with black beans and avocado
- Pasta with lentil Bolognese

Step 2: Prep Staples in Bulk

- Cook a large pot of beans or lentils
- Roast a tray of mixed veggies
- Make a big batch of quinoa or rice
- Prepare sauces (tahini dressing, tomato sauce, hummus)

These staples can be mixed and matched throughout the week.

Step 3: Grocery Shopping List Framework

- **Proteins:** lentils, chickpeas, tofu, tempeh, seitan
- **Grains:** oats, rice, quinoa, whole-wheat bread/pasta
- **Veggies:** leafy greens, cruciferous veggies, root veggies
- **Fruits:** bananas, apples, berries, oranges
- **Fats:** nuts, seeds, avocado, olive oil
- **Extras:** herbs, spices, nutritional yeast, plant-based milk

3. Tracking Nutrition (Without Obsession)

One common concern is missing nutrients. While most needs can be met through variety, a little tracking especially at the beginning can give peace of mind.

Nutrients to Prioritize Long-Term

- **Vitamin B12:** Supplement (daily or weekly).
- **Vitamin D:** From sunlight or supplement if needed.
- **Omega-3s:** Flax, chia, hemp, walnuts, or algae oil.
- **Iron & Zinc:** Lentils, beans, pumpkin seeds, fortified cereals.
- **Calcium:** Fortified plant milk, tofu, greens, almonds.
- **Protein:** Variety of legumes, soy products, grains, and nuts.

Tools for Tracking

- Apps like Cronometer or MyFitnessPal can help ensure balance, especially in the first few months.
- Once you're familiar with portions and sources, tracking often becomes unnecessary.

4. Building Long-Term Habits

The most successful long-term vegans share one trait: they've built habits that stick, even during busy times.

Keystone Habits

- **Sunday Prep:** A few hours of batch cooking make weekdays easier.
- **Always Stock Snacks:** Keep nuts, fruit, or protein bars handy.
- **Learn 5 "Lazy Meals":** Quick go-to meals you can make in 10 minutes (like hummus wraps, bean burritos, or tofu stir-fry).

- **Restaurant Routine:** Always scan menus ahead of time or have a go-to vegan-friendly place in mind.

5. Handling Setbacks Without Quitting

Long-term sustainability doesn't mean never slipping. It means learning how to bounce back.

- If you eat something non-vegan by mistake → Note it, move on.
- If you feel bored → Try one new recipe or cuisine each week.
- If you feel low-energy → Reassess protein, iron, and sleep habits.
- If social pressure wears you down → Reconnect with your health goals and your "why."

Remember: It's not about being perfect; it's about being consistent over time.

6. Creating Joy, Not Just Discipline

For a diet to last, it has to bring you joy. That means experimenting, indulging sometimes, and finding meals you *look forward* to.

- Try vegan versions of your favorite comfort foods (pizza, burgers, lasagna).
- Explore international cuisines many are naturally plant-based.
- Celebrate milestones (30 days, 6 months, 1 year) with new recipes or dining experiences.

Takeaway: Structure Creates Freedom

When you build routines, meal systems, and healthy habits, veganism stops being "something you do" and becomes "who you are." Instead of making dozens of food decisions daily, you'll have a reliable structure that supports your health while leaving room for joy and spontaneity.

Long-term success doesn't come from willpower alone it comes from structure. And once that structure is in place, the lifestyle becomes effortless.

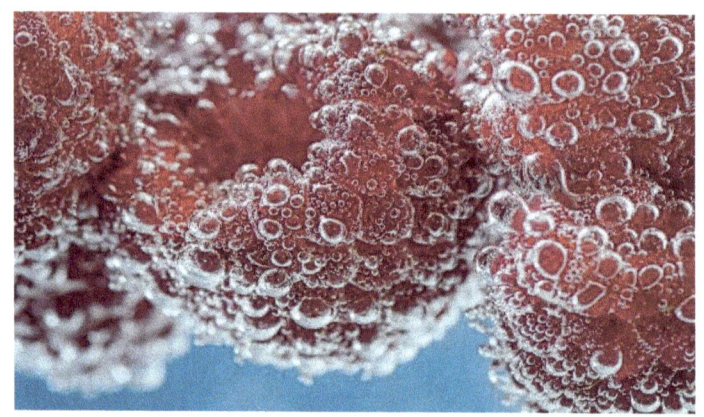

Chapter 10: Beyond the Plate

At first, going vegan for health may feel like a purely physical decision: lower cholesterol, more energy, healthier weight. But as the weeks stretch into months, something remarkable begins to happen. The change isn't just in your body it's in your mind, your emotions, and your sense of self.

This chapter is about those deeper ripples. What happens when food becomes more than fuel, and when eating plants connects you to something bigger than just your health?

The Quiet Mind

Many people describe an unexpected side effect of going plant-based: a sense of mental clarity.

When *Leah*, a 29-year-old nurse, shifted her diet, she noticed she no longer had the heavy "fog" after lunch. She could focus through her shifts, stay present with patients, and even felt less irritable at home.

Science can explain some of this balanced blood sugar, anti-inflammatory foods, steady energy but part of it is more subtle. When your body is nourished with clean, vibrant foods, your mind often feels lighter too.

It's like static clears from the radio, and you can finally hear yourself again.

The Emotional Shift

Food is deeply emotional. For years, many of us use it as comfort, distraction, or a way to numb stress. When you change your diet intentionally, you also change your relationship with yourself.

David, a 50-year-old father, admitted:

"I used to eat whatever was in front of me. Going vegan forced me to pause and actually think: what am I putting into my body, and why?"

This awareness spills into other areas of life. You may notice yourself slowing down, becoming more intentional, and treating your body with care rather than punishment.

Food stops being just something you consume. It becomes a daily act of self-respect.

Identity and Alignment

There's a unique empowerment that comes from saying: *I am choosing this.*

Unlike a temporary diet, going vegan for health is an identity shift. You're no longer passively following old habits you're consciously living in a way that aligns with your values and goals.

That alignment creates inner peace. Every meal becomes a statement: *I value my health. I choose energy. I choose life.*

For many, this sense of alignment spreads into other choices: exercising more, sleeping better, handling stress with mindfulness instead of food. The plate becomes a mirror for the person you want to be.

Connection to Something Larger

Even if you start veganism purely for health, it's hard not to notice the ripple effects. You become more aware of where food comes from the soil, the farmers, the ecosystems that sustain us.

Eating plants can feel grounding, even spiritual. It's a way of connecting to cycles of nature, to the seasons, to life itself.

Maria, a 34-year-old artist, shared:

"I didn't expect to feel so connected. When I cook beans or chop vegetables, I feel like I'm participating in something ancient and human — the way food was always meant to nourish us."

Health may be the doorway, but connection is the gift waiting on the other side.

The Ripple Effect on Others

Perhaps the most profound change happens not just in you, but in those around you.

When you live with intention, people notice. Your energy, your resilience, your choices quietly inspire others friends, family, even coworkers.

Remember Daniel from Chapter 8? His coworkers teased him at first, but months later, some of them asked for recipes. His wife began adding more vegetables to her own meals. Without preaching or pushing, he created change simply by being an example.

The food on your plate becomes more than nutrition. It becomes a ripple of health that spreads outward.

Takeaway: A Way of Being

What begins as a diet often becomes a way of being. Veganism for health isn't just about cholesterol or weight it's about clarity, alignment, connection, and the quiet confidence that comes from living in tune with your values.

It's proof that the choices we make at the table are never just physical. They shape our minds, our emotions, and even the people around us.

When you go beyond the plate, you discover that food is not just fuel it's a path toward becoming more fully alive.

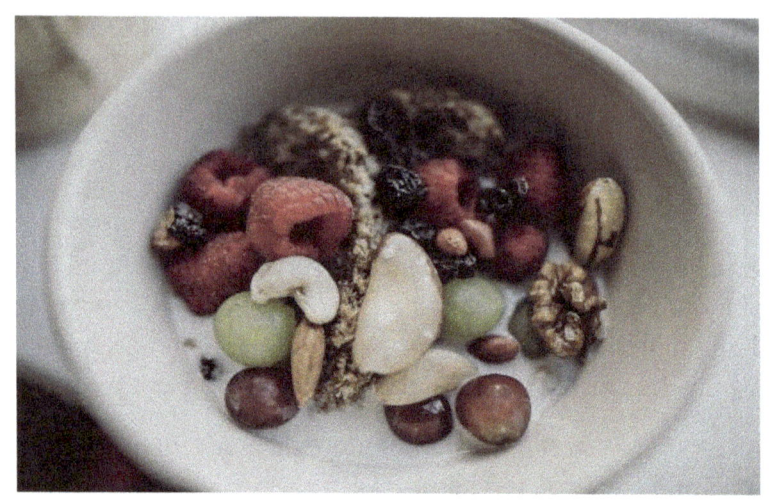

Chapter 11: Plant-based Lifestyle

You've taken a journey from learning the science of plant-based health, to navigating your first 30 days, to facing challenges, to finding deeper meaning beyond the plate. By now, you can see that going vegan for health isn't just about what you *don't* eat it's about what you gain.

Energy. Clarity. Confidence. A sense of alignment between who you want to be and how you live.

This Is Not the End It's the Beginning

The chapters you've read aren't meant to be rules written in stone. They're a starting point a foundation you can build on, adjust, and personalize.

Your vegan journey will not be perfect. There will be slip-ups, cravings, and social challenges. But here's the truth: perfection isn't the goal. Consistency is. Each meal is a chance to nourish yourself, to reaffirm your choice, and to take one more step toward the healthiest version of you.

Why You Matters Most

Remember why you started. Maybe it was your health, your energy, your family, or a warning from your doctor. That "why" is your compass. Whenever you feel uncertain, return to it.

The deeper you connect to your "why," the stronger your resolve becomes.

Small Steps Lead to Big Change

Don't underestimate the power of small, steady steps.

- Choosing beans instead of beef at dinner.
- Saying yes to fruit instead of dessert one night.
- Trying a new recipe with your family.

Over time, these tiny shifts add up. They reshape your habits, your body, and your life. A year from now, you'll look back and be amazed at how far you've come.

You Are Part of Something Bigger

Even if you began this journey for your own health, your choice carries ripples beyond yourself. You're showing your loved ones that change is possible. You're proving that it's never too late to start again. You're embodying the idea that food can be medicine, joy, and self-respect all at once.

Your journey may even inspire others to take their own first step.

The Power of Small Steps

Change doesn't happen in a giant leap. It happens in small, consistent steps:

- Choosing oatmeal over eggs.
- Packing a plant-based lunch instead of grabbing fast food.
- Trying one new recipe a week.

These steps add up. They transform your habits, your body, and your mindset. One day, you'll look back and realize how far you've come and you'll be grateful you started.

You're Not Alone

I used to think I had to do it all by myself. But I learned that community matters. Find people online or in person who share your journey. Ask questions. Swap recipes. Celebrate wins, no matter how small.

And remember: by choosing this path, you're also inspiring others. Without even realizing it, you're becoming an example of what's possible.

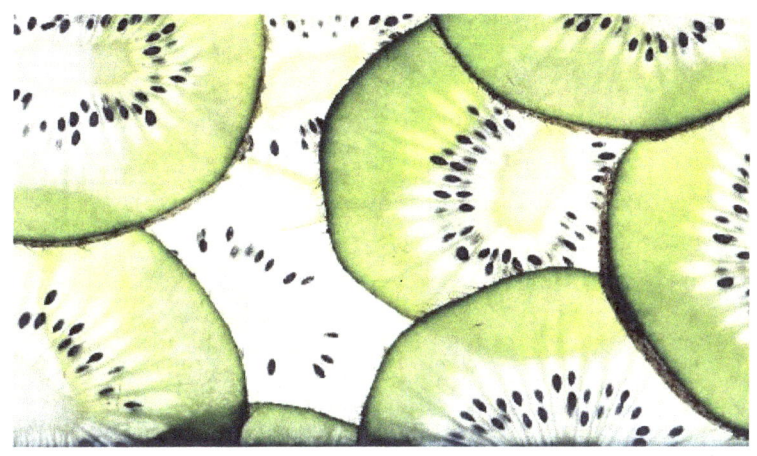

Chapter 12: Conclusion & Resources

"Every new beginning comes from some other beginning's end."

- Seneca

When I first made the choice to embrace a vegan lifestyle, I thought it was simply about food. But it became so much more. It became about life itself.

The benefits have been undeniable: improved energy, stabilized blood pressure, better digestion, and a renewed sense of vitality. But beyond the physical, I gained something even more valuable peace of mind. I now live knowing that I am actively protecting my health and investing in my future.

If you are considering this journey, I want you to know that it is possible. You don't need to be perfect, and you don't have to do it overnight. Begin with one plant-based meal. Learn as you go. Celebrate small victories. Over time, these small steps add up to profound transformation.

This book is not the end of my story but the beginning of a lifelong commitment. My hope is that it becomes a stepping stone for you a guide, a source of encouragement, and a reminder that thriving is within your reach. -Dr. Sandra Michael-Johnson

🌱 **Recommended Resources for Your Journey:**

- **Books**: *How Not to Die* by Michael Greger, *The China Study* by T. Colin Campbell, *Prevent and Reverse Heart Disease* by Caldwell Esselstyn

- **Websites**: NutritionFacts.org, ForksOverKnives.com, HappyCow.net

- **Documentaries**: *Forks Over Knives*, *The Game Changers*, *What the Health*

Your journey is uniquely yours, but remember: you are not alone. Countless others have walked this path, and you have an entire community waiting to support you.

Here's to your health, your healing, and you're thriving on plants.

Discover the Healing Power of Plants

After years of long hours and the stress of running national healthcare agencies, Dr. Sandra Michael-Johnson faced a wake-up call: fatigue and a hypertension scare. Determined to reclaim her health, she turned to a plant-based lifestyle and found transformation.

In *Thriving on Plants: A Journey to Health and Healing Through Vegan Living*, Dr. Michael-Johnson shares her personal story alongside practical guidance to help you take control of your health. Through a blend of science, personal experience, and compassion, she shows how food can be both medicine and joy.

Inside, you'll find:

- The health benefits of a vegan lifestyle explained in clear, accessible language
- Strategies for overcoming common challenges in transitioning to plant-based eating
- A 7-day meal plan and delicious starter recipes
- Reflections to inspire strength, resilience, and self-care

Whether you are curious, just starting out, or seeking long-term wellness, this book offers encouragement and practical tools to help you thrive—body, mind, and spirit—on plants.

🌍 Why Veganism Matters: The Bigger Picture

Adopting a vegan lifestyle isn't just about diet—it's about transformation. It reshapes our health, protects the planet, saves lives, and promotes compassion. Below are some striking insights and statistics that highlight the urgency and importance of veganism.

🌱 For Health

- A plant-based diet is associated with a **25% lower risk of ischemic heart disease** (Journal of the American Heart Association, 2021).
- Vegans typically have **lower BMIs, cholesterol levels, and blood pressure** compared to omnivores (British Dietetic Association, 2020).
- Studies show that replacing animal protein with plant protein can **reduce overall mortality risk by 10%** (JAMA Internal Medicine, 2020).
- High fiber intake from plants supports gut health, immune function, and lowers risk of colorectal cancer.

🌍 For the Planet

- If everyone adopted a vegan diet, global food-related emissions could drop by **up to 70% by 2050** (Oxford University, 2016).
- Livestock production accounts for **nearly 80% of global deforestation**, much of it in the Amazon rainforest (World Bank).
- Producing 1 pound of beef requires **1,800 gallons of water**, while 1 pound of lentils needs only **75 gallons** (Water Footprint Network).
- Switching to a vegan diet could save **6 million lives per year** and cut healthcare costs by **$1.5 trillion annually** (Proceedings of the National Academy of Sciences, 2016).

🐾 For Animals

- Each year, more than **70 billion land animals** and over **1 trillion sea animals** are killed for food (FAO & Fish count).
- In the U.S. alone, **9 billion chickens** are slaughtered annually, often in overcrowded, inhumane conditions.
- Factory farming confines animals in small cages or pens, depriving them of natural behaviors. Veganism directly challenges this system.
- By going vegan, one person can save **over 200 animals each year**—a lifetime impact that can reach thousands of lives spared.

🌐 For Global Justice

- Nearly **820 million people worldwide are undernourished**, while one-third of global grain production is used to feed livestock, not people (FAO).
- Shifting to plant-based diets would free vast amounts of land and crops, potentially helping to feed the growing population sustainably.
- Veganism supports global food equity by prioritizing efficient use of resources to nourish people, not livestock.

💡 The Takeaway

Veganism is one of the **most powerful lifestyle choices** you can make:

- For **your body** → lower disease risk, more vitality, longer life.
- For **the Earth** → reduced emissions, water savings, preserved forests.
- For **animals** → freedom from suffering, compassion, and dignity.
- For **society** → justice, sustainability, and hope for future generations.

Every meal is a vote—for health, for the planet, and for kindness.

- killed for food each year worldwide (FAO).
- Every person who adopts a vegan lifestyle spare **about 200 animals per year** (Humane Society estimates).

Personal Transformation Stories

🌱 My Journey to Thriving on Plants

For years, I thought health was only about exercise and moderation, but I didn't realize the profound impact food has on every part of our lives from physical vitality to mental clarity. When I transitioned to a plant-based lifestyle, I wasn't just changing what was on my plate I was rewriting my relationship with food, with my body, and with the planet.

At first, it was intimidating. Family dinners, restaurant menus, and even grocery aisles felt unfamiliar. But soon, something remarkable happened: I discovered flavors, colors, and textures I had overlooked my whole life. Meals became not just fuel, but a celebration.

The benefits followed quickly: more energy in the mornings, improved digestion, clearer skin, and a deep sense of alignment with my values. For me, veganism became more than a diet it became a way of living that honored both my health and the wellbeing of the world around me.

☀ Case Study 1: Maya's Journey from Fatigue to Energy

Maya, a busy teacher, struggled with constant fatigue and frequent colds. She decided to experiment with plant-based eating for 30 days. Within weeks, her energy levels skyrocketed. Instead of relying on coffee to get through her afternoons, she felt naturally alert and focused. The biggest surprise for Maya? Her chronic migraines, which had plagued her for years, began to fade. She now calls veganism her "energy medicine."

☀ Case Study 2: Daniel's Story of Compassion and Clarity

Daniel, a lifelong foodie, initially resisted veganism, thinking it would limit his love for cooking. But after watching a documentary on animal welfare, he decided to give it a try. To his amazement, he discovered a new world of creativity in the kitchen. He began experimenting with global vegan dishes, from Thai curries to Italian pastas. Not only did his health markers improve lower cholesterol and weight loss but he also found peace in knowing his meals aligned with his compassion for animals.

Practical How-To Guides

🛒 Pantry Makeover: Building a Vegan-Friendly Kitchen

Transitioning begins in your pantry. A well-stocked kitchen makes plant-based cooking easy and stress-free.

Step 1: Clear the Clutter

- Remove processed snacks, meat products, dairy, and items high in refined sugar.
- Donate unopened non-vegan foods to local shelters.

Step 2: Add the Essentials

- **Proteins**: Lentils, chickpeas, black beans, tofu, tempeh, quinoa.
- **Grains**: Brown rice, oats, bulgur, barley, couscous, whole wheat pasta.
- **Nuts & Seeds**: Almonds, walnuts, chia, flax, sunflower, hemp seeds.
- **Dairy Alternatives**: Plant-based milks (oat, soy, almond, cashew), coconut yogurt, vegan cheese.
- **Flavor Boosters**: Nutritional yeast, miso paste, tahini, spices, fresh herbs.

Step 3: Fresh Additions

- Stock up on colorful produce: leafy greens, cruciferous vegetables, berries, root veggies, and seasonal fruits.

🛍 Smart Shopping Tips

- **Shop the perimeter** of the grocery store — produce, grains, beans, and nuts are often found here.
- **Read labels carefully**: animal products may hide under names like casein, whey, gelatin, or rennet.
- **Buy in bulk**: beans, rice, oats, and nuts are often cheaper and reduce packaging waste.
- **Seasonal & local**: Farmers' markets offer fresh, affordable, and sustainable produce.

🍽 Eating Out as a Vegan

- **Research ahead**: Look up menus online before going to restaurants.
- **Ask kindly**: Most chefs are happy to modify dishes if you request.
- **Go global**: Many international cuisines naturally feature vegan options (Indian, Ethiopian, Thai, Mediterranean).
- **Bring a backup**: Keep nuts, dried fruit, or vegan protein bars handy when traveling.

📅 Transition Plan: A 4-Week Guide

Week 1: Remove red meat, add one plant-based meal daily.
Week 2: Eliminate poultry, increase legumes and whole grains.
Week 3: Replace dairy with plant alternatives, try vegan baking.
Week 4: Remove fish/eggs, fully transition to plant-based eating.

👉 Tip: Don't stress about perfection every plant-based choice makes an impact.

The Science of Veganism

℞ Health Benefits of Veganism

1. Heart Health

- Studies show that plant-based diets lower LDL ("bad") cholesterol and reduce the risk of heart disease by up to **32%**.
- Diets high in fiber and antioxidants from fruits, vegetables, and legumes improve blood pressure and circulation.

2. Diabetes & Blood Sugar

- Vegans have a **50–78% lower risk** of developing type 2 diabetes.
- Plant foods improve insulin sensitivity and stabilize blood sugar.

3. Cancer Prevention

- The World Health Organization (WHO) lists processed meats as carcinogenic.
- Diets rich in fiber, phytonutrients, and antioxidants found in plants may lower the risk of colon, breast, and prostate cancer.

4. Weight Management

- Vegans typically have lower body mass indexes (BMIs).
- High-fiber foods create satiety, reducing overeating.

5. Longevity & Quality of Life

- Blue Zone research (world regions with the longest-living people) shows heavy reliance on plant-based diets.

- Vegan diets reduce chronic inflammation, supporting healthy aging.

🌍 Environmental Impact of Veganism

1. Carbon Footprint

- Animal agriculture contributes nearly **15% of global greenhouse gas emissions**.
- A vegan diet can reduce your food-related carbon footprint by **50% or more**.

2. Land Use

- 77% of global farmland is used for livestock, yet it only produces 18% of calories consumed worldwide.
- If everyone shifted to plant-based diets, we could free up land the size of Africa.

3. Water Usage

- It takes **1,800 gallons of water** to produce 1 pound of beef.
- By contrast, producing 1 pound of lentils requires only **200 gallons**.

4. Biodiversity

- Deforestation for animal farming destroys ecosystems.
- Eating plants supports habitat conservation and protects endangered species.

🐄 Ethical & Social Justice Perspective

- **Animal Welfare**: Billions of animals are raised and killed in factory farms annually under inhumane conditions. Veganism reduces demand for this suffering.
- **Global Hunger**: 70% of crops grown globally are fed to livestock instead of humans. Shifting food systems toward plants could help alleviate world hunger.
- **Social Justice**: Communities near factory farms face pollution, poor air quality, and contaminated water. A plant-based food system can reduce these inequities.

As an appreciation of you embarking on your new lifestyle, I have shared some of my favorite recipes.

NOW IT'S TIME TO ENJOY SOME OF MY FAVORITE RECIPES.

Recipes for Thriving Throughout Your Vegan Journey

Recipes: these are some recipes I've enjoyed throughout my vegan journey. May you savor the forty plus recipes that includes breakfast, lunch, dinner, desserts, and snacks.

🌊 Breakfast – Energizing Overnight Oats

Ingredients:

- ½ cup rolled oats
- 1 cup unsweetened almond milk
- 1 Tbsp chia seeds
- 1 tsp cinnamon
- ½ cup mixed berries
- 1 tsp maple syrup (optional)

Instructions:

1. Combine oats, almond milk, chia seeds, and cinnamon in a jar.
2. Stir, cover, and refrigerate overnight.
3. In the morning, top with berries and a drizzle of maple syrup.

Energizing Overnight Oats

Ingredients:

- ½ cup rolled oats
- 1 cup unsweetened almond milk
- 1 Tbsp chia seeds
- 1 tsp cinnamon
- ½ cup mixed berries
- 1 tsp maple syrup (optional)

Instructions:

1. Combine oats, almond milk, chia seeds, and cinnamon in a jar.
2. Stir, cover, and refrigerate overnight.
3. Top with berries and maple syrup before serving.

✦ *Health Tip:* Rich in fiber and antioxidants, this keeps energy levels steady all morning.

Tofu Scramble with Spinach & Peppers

Ingredients:

- 1 block firm tofu, crumbled
- 1 Tbsp olive oil
- 1 cup fresh spinach
- ½ cup chopped bell peppers
- ½ tsp turmeric
- Salt & black pepper to taste

Instructions:

1. Heat oil in a skillet, add crumbled tofu.
2. Season with turmeric, salt, and pepper.
3. Stir in spinach and peppers; cook until tender.

✧ *Health Tip:* A protein-rich alternative to scrambled eggs, packed with iron and calcium.

Savory Tofu Scramble

Prep Time: 5 min | **Cook Time:** 10 min | **Servings:** 2 | **Nutrition (per serving):** Calories: 210 | Protein: 18 g | Fat: 12 g | Carbs: 10 g

Ingredients:

- 1 block firm tofu, crumbled
- 1 tbsp olive oil
- ½ onion, diced
- 1 bell pepper, diced
- 1 tsp turmeric
- 1 tsp nutritional yeast
- Salt and pepper to taste
- Fresh parsley, chopped

Instructions:

1. Heat olive oil in a skillet over medium heat. Sauté onion and bell pepper until soft.
2. Add crumbled tofu, turmeric, nutritional yeast, salt, and pepper. Cook 5–7 minutes, stirring frequently.
3. Garnish with parsley and serve warm.

Banana Pancakes with Maple Drizzle

Ingredients:

- 1 ripe banana (mashed)
- 1 cup whole wheat flour
- 1 tsp baking powder
- 1 cup almond milk
- 1 tsp vanilla extract
- Maple syrup, for serving

Instructions:

1. Mix mashed banana, almond milk, and vanilla.
2. Add flour and baking powder, whisk until smooth.
3. Cook on a greased skillet until golden.
4. Serve with maple syrup.

✨ *Health Tip:* Naturally sweetened with banana, these pancakes are wholesome and satisfying.

Fluffy Vegan Pancakes

Prep Time: 10 min | **Cook Time:** 15 min | **Servings:** 4 | **Nutrition (per serving):** Calories: 250 | Protein: 6 g | Fat: 6 g | Carbs: 42 g

Ingredients:

- 1 cup all-purpose flour
- 2 tbsp sugar
- 2 tsp baking powder
- ¼ tsp salt

- 1 cup almond milk
- 2 tbsp coconut oil, melted
- 1 tsp vanilla extract

Instructions:

1. In a bowl, mix flour, sugar, baking powder, and salt.
2. Stir in almond milk, coconut oil, and vanilla until smooth.
3. Heat a non-stick skillet over medium heat. Pour ¼ cup batter per pancake. Cook until bubbles form, then flip and cook 2–3 minutes more.
4. Serve with maple syrup and fresh fruit.

Tropical Smoothie Bowl

Prep Time: 10 min | **Cook Time:** 0 min | **Servings:** 2 | **Nutrition (per serving):** Calories: 320 | Protein: 6 g | Fat: 8 g | Carbs: 58 g

Ingredients:

- 1 banana, frozen
- 1 cup mango chunks, frozen
- ½ cup pineapple chunks, frozen
- ½ cup unsweetened almond milk
- 1 tbsp chia seeds
- ¼ cup granola (for topping)
- Fresh berries and coconut flakes (for topping)

Instructions:

1. Blend banana, mango, pineapple, and almond milk until smooth.

2. Pour into bowls. Sprinkle chia seeds, granola, berries, and coconut flakes on top.
3. Serve immediately for a refreshing breakfast boost.

Overnight Oats with Berries

Prep Time: 5 min | **Cook Time:** 0 min | **Servings:** 2 | **Nutrition (per serving):** Calories: 300 | Protein: 8 g | Fat: 7 g | Carbs: 52 g

Ingredients:

- 1 cup rolled oats
- 1 cup almond milk
- 2 tbsp chia seeds
- 1 tbsp maple syrup
- ½ tsp vanilla extract
- ½ cup mixed berries

Instructions:

1. Combine oats, almond milk, chia seeds, maple syrup, and vanilla in a jar or bowl.
2. Refrigerate overnight.
3. Top with berries before serving.

Avocado Toast with Chickpeas

Prep Time: 10 min | **Cook Time:** 5 min | **Servings:** 2 | **Nutrition (per serving):** Calories: 280 | Protein: 10 g | Fat: 14 g | Carbs: 30 g

Ingredients:

- 4 slices whole-grain bread, toasted
- 1 ripe avocado

- ½ cup chickpeas, mashed
- 1 tsp lemon juice
- Salt and pepper to taste
- Red pepper flakes (optional)

Instructions:

1. Mash avocado with lemon juice, salt, and pepper.
2. Spread avocado on toasted bread.
3. Top with mashed chickpeas and a sprinkle of red pepper flakes

Lunch Recipes

Quinoa & Roasted Veggie Salad

Prep Time: 15 min | **Cook Time:** 30 min | **Servings:** 2 | **Nutrition (per serving):** Calories: 420 | Protein: 12 g | Fat: 14 g | Carbs: 62 g

Ingredients:

- 1 cup quinoa, rinsed
- 2 cups water or vegetable broth
- 1 zucchini, sliced
- 1 red bell pepper, chopped
- 1 cup broccoli florets
- 2 tbsp olive oil
- 1 tsp smoked paprika
- Salt and pepper to taste
- ¼ cup tahini
- 2 tbsp lemon juice
- 1 tbsp maple syrup
- Water to thin

Instructions:

1. Preheat oven to 400°F (200°C). Toss zucchini, bell pepper, and broccoli with olive oil, smoked paprika, salt, and pepper. Roast 20–25 minutes.
2. Cook quinoa with water or broth according to package instructions.
3. Whisk tahini, lemon juice, maple syrup, and water to make dressing.

4. Serve roasted veggies over quinoa and drizzle with dressing.

Chickpea Salad Sandwich

Prep Time: 10 min | **Cook Time:** 0 min | **Servings:** 2 | **Nutrition (per serving):** Calories: 330 | Protein: 12 g | Fat: 11 g | Carbs: 42 g

Ingredients:

- 1 can chickpeas, drained and mashed
- 2 tbsp vegan mayo
- 1 tsp Dijon mustard
- ½ tsp garlic powder
- Salt and pepper to taste
- 4 slices whole-grain bread
- Lettuce, tomato, and cucumber slices

Instructions:

1. In a bowl, mix mashed chickpeas, vegan mayo, Dijon mustard, garlic powder, salt, and pepper.
2. Spread mixture on bread slices. Top with lettuce, tomato, and cucumber.
3. Serve immediately or wrap for lunch on the go.

Rainbow Quinoa Power Salad

Serves: 4 | **Prep Time:** 20 min | **Cook Time:** 15 min

Ingredients

- 1 cup quinoa, rinsed
- 2 cups vegetable broth
- 1 cup cherry tomatoes, halved

- 1 cucumber, diced
- 1 yellow bell pepper, diced
- 1 cup shredded carrots
- 1 cup baby spinach or arugula
- ¼ cup red onion, finely chopped
- ¼ cup fresh parsley, chopped

Dressing

- 3 tbsp olive oil
- 2 tbsp lemon juice
- 1 tbsp apple cider vinegar
- 1 tsp maple syrup
- Salt & pepper to taste

Instructions

1. Cook quinoa in vegetable broth until fluffy; let cool.
2. In a large bowl, combine quinoa, veggies, and parsley.
3. Whisk dressing ingredients and pour over salad.
4. Toss gently and serve chilled.

✨ *A protein-packed salad that's as colorful as it is nutritious.*

Creamy Avocado Kale Salad

Serves: 2–3 | **Prep Time:** 15 min

Ingredients

- 1 large bunch kale, stems removed, leaves chopped
- 1 avocado, ripe
- 2 tbsp lemon juice
- 1 tbsp tahini
- 1 tsp Dijon mustard

- 1 clove garlic, minced
- ¼ cup sunflower seeds or pumpkin seeds
- ¼ cup dried cranberries

Instructions

1. In a large bowl, mash avocado with lemon juice, tahini, mustard, and garlic until creamy.
2. Add kale and massage dressing into the leaves for 2–3 minutes to soften.
3. Top with seeds and cranberries before serving.

✨ *A nutrient-dense, iron-rich salad with natural creaminess from avocado.*

Mediterranean Chickpea Salad

Serves: 4 | **Prep Time:** 10 min

Ingredients

- 2 cans chickpeas, drained and rinsed
- 1 cucumber, diced
- 1 cup cherry tomatoes, halved
- ½ red onion, finely diced
- ¼ cup kalamata olives, sliced
- ¼ cup fresh parsley, chopped

Dressing

- 3 tbsp extra-virgin olive oil
- 2 tbsp red wine vinegar
- 1 tsp oregano
- Salt & pepper to taste

Instructions

1. Combine chickpeas, cucumber, tomatoes, onion, olives, and parsley.
2. Whisk dressing ingredients and toss with salad.
3. Serve immediately or chill for 1 hour for deeper flavor.

✨ *A light yet filling salad inspired by the Mediterranean diet.*

Mango Black Bean Fiesta Salad

Serves: 4 | **Prep Time:** 15 min

Ingredients

- 1 can black beans, drained and rinsed
- 1 ripe mango, diced
- 1 red bell pepper, diced
- 1 cup corn (fresh or frozen, thawed)
- ¼ cup red onion, diced
- ¼ cup cilantro, chopped

Dressing

- 2 tbsp lime juice
- 2 tbsp olive oil
- 1 tsp agave or maple syrup
- ½ tsp chili powder
- Salt to taste

Instructions

1. Mix black beans, mango, pepper, corn, onion, and cilantro in a bowl.
2. In a small jar, shake together dressing ingredients.

3. Pour over salad and toss well.

✨ *Sweet, tangy, and slightly spicy – a tropical twist on bean salad.*

Roasted Sweet Potato & Arugula Salad

Serves: 3–4 | **Prep Time:** 10 min | **Cook Time:** 25 min

Ingredients

- 2 medium sweet potatoes, cubed
- 1 tbsp olive oil
- 1 tsp smoked paprika
- 4 cups arugula
- ¼ cup walnuts, toasted
- ¼ cup dried cranberries
- 2 tbsp pumpkin seeds

Dressing

- 3 tbsp balsamic vinegar
- 2 tbsp olive oil
- 1 tsp Dijon mustard
- 1 tsp maple syrup
- Salt & pepper to taste

Instructions

1. Toss sweet potatoes with olive oil and paprika; roast at 400°F (200°C) for 25 min.
2. In a large bowl, combine arugula, walnuts, cranberries, and pumpkin seeds.
3. Add roasted sweet potatoes.
4. Drizzle with balsamic dressing and serve warm.

✦ A hearty, antioxidant-rich salad perfect for a main course.

Avocado & Black Bean Salad

Prep Time: 10 min | **Cook Time:** 0 min | **Servings:** 2 | **Nutrition (per serving):** Calories: 360 | Protein: 12 g | Fat: 18 g | Carbs: 40 g

Ingredients:

- 1 can black beans, drained and rinsed
- 1 avocado, diced
- 1 cup cherry tomatoes, halved
- ½ red onion, diced
- 2 tbsp lime juice
- Salt and pepper to taste
- Fresh cilantro for garnish

Instructions:

1. In a bowl, mix black beans, avocado, tomatoes, and onion.
2. Drizzle with lime juice and season with salt and pepper.
3. Garnish with cilantro and serve chilled.

Vegan Pasta Récipes

🌿 Creamy Cashew Alfredo Pasta

Ingredients

- 12 oz whole wheat fettuccine
- 1 cup raw cashews (soaked 4 hours)
- 2 cloves garlic
- 1 cup unsweetened almond milk
- 2 tbsp nutritional yeast
- 1 tbsp lemon juice
- Salt & pepper to taste
- Fresh parsley for garnish

Instructions

1. Cook pasta according to package directions.
2. Blend soaked cashews, garlic, almond milk, nutritional yeast, lemon juice, salt, and pepper until creamy.
3. Drain pasta and toss with sauce.
4. Garnish with parsley and serve warm.

🍅 Roasted Tomato & Basil Penne

Ingredients

- 12 oz penne pasta
- 2 cups cherry tomatoes, halved
- 3 tbsp olive oil
- 3 garlic cloves, minced
- 1 cup fresh basil leaves
- Salt & pepper to taste

Instructions

1. Roast cherry tomatoes with olive oil, garlic, salt, and pepper at 400°F for 20 minutes.
2. Cook penne until al dente.
3. Toss pasta with roasted tomatoes and basil.
4. Drizzle with extra olive oil before serving.

Pesto Pasta with Spinach & Walnuts

Ingredients

- 12 oz spaghetti or linguine
- 2 cups fresh spinach
- 1 cup basil leaves
- ½ cup walnuts
- 2 tbsp nutritional yeast
- ¼ cup olive oil
- 2 tbsp lemon juice
- Salt to taste

Instructions

1. Blend spinach, basil, walnuts, nutritional yeast, olive oil, lemon juice, and salt into pesto.
2. Cook pasta and toss with pesto sauce.
3. Top with extra walnuts for crunch.

Spicy Arrabbiata Pasta

Ingredients

- 12 oz rigatoni or penne
- 2 tbsp olive oil
- 4 garlic cloves, minced

- ½ tsp red pepper flakes (adjust to taste)
- 2 cups crushed tomatoes
- 1 tsp oregano
- Fresh parsley

Instructions

1. Heat olive oil, sauté garlic and red pepper flakes.
2. Add crushed tomatoes and oregano, simmer 15 minutes.
3. Cook pasta and mix with sauce.
4. Top with parsley before serving.

🍄 Mushroom & Spinach Creamy Pasta

Ingredients

- 12 oz fusilli pasta
- 2 cups mushrooms, sliced
- 3 cups spinach
- 1 cup oat milk
- 1 tbsp flour
- 2 tbsp olive oil
- Salt & pepper

Instructions

1. Cook pasta.
2. In a pan, sauté mushrooms in olive oil until golden. Add spinach.
3. Whisk flour into oat milk and pour into pan. Cook until creamy.
4. Toss pasta with sauce. Season and serve warm.

✨ These recipes bring variety creamy, fresh, spicy, and wholesome pasta options all fully vegan and health-focused.

Creamy Cashew Alfredo Pasta

Prep Time: 10 min | **Cook Time:** 15 min | **Servings:** 4

Ingredients:

- 12 oz fettuccine or pasta of choice
- 1 cup raw cashews, soaked 2 hours
- 1 cup unsweetened almond milk
- 2 tbsp nutritional yeast
- 2 garlic cloves
- 1 tsp lemon juice
- Salt and pepper to taste
- Fresh parsley for garnish

Instructions:

1. Cook pasta according to package instructions. Drain and set aside.
2. Blend-soaked cashews, almond milk, nutritional yeast, garlic, and lemon juice until smooth.
3. Pour sauce into a pan and warm over medium heat, seasoning with salt and pepper.
4. Toss pasta in sauce and garnish with parsley. Serve immediately.

Vegan Lentil Soup

Prep Time: 10 min | **Cook Time:** 30 min | **Servings:** 4 | **Nutrition (per serving):** Calories: 220 | Protein: 12 g | Fat: 5 g | Carbs: 35 g

Ingredients:

- 1 cup red lentils, rinsed

- 1 tbsp olive oil
- 1 onion, chopped
- 2 garlic cloves, minced
- 2 carrots, chopped
- 2 celery stalks, chopped
- 1 can (14 oz) diced tomatoes
- 4 cups vegetable broth
- 1 tsp cumin
- ½ tsp paprika
- Salt and pepper to taste

Instructions:

1. Heat olive oil in a pot over medium heat. Sauté onion, garlic, carrots, and celery 5 minutes.
2. Add lentils, tomatoes, broth, cumin, paprika, salt, and pepper.
3. Bring to boil, then simmer 20 minutes until lentils are tender.
4. Serve warm, garnished with fresh herbs if desired.

Raw Energy Balls

Prep Time: 15 min | **Cook Time:** 0 min | **Servings:** 12 balls | **Nutrition (per ball):** Calories: 110 | Protein: 3 g | Fat: 6 g | Carbs: 12 g

Ingredients:

- 1 cup dates, pitted
- ½ cup almonds
- ¼ cup shredded coconut

- 2 tbsp cocoa powder
- 1 tbsp chia seeds

Instructions:

1. Blend all ingredients in a food processor until sticky and well combined.
2. Roll into 12 small balls.
3. Store in the fridge for a quick snack.

Coconut Rice Pudding

Prep Time: 5 min | **Cook Time:** 25 min | **Servings:** 4 | **Nutrition (per serving):** Calories: 250 | Protein: 4 g | Fat: 8 g | Carbs: 40 g

Ingredients:

- 1 cup jasmine rice
- 2 cups coconut milk
- ¼ cup maple syrup
- 1 tsp vanilla extract
- Pinch of salt
- Toasted coconut or berries for topping

Instructions:

1. Combine rice, coconut milk, maple syrup, vanilla, and salt in a saucepan.
2. Bring to a simmer and cook 20–25 minutes until rice is tender, stirring occasionally.
3. Serve warm or chilled, topped with toasted coconut or berries.

Berry Crumble

Prep Time: 10 min | **Cook Time:** 30 min | **Servings:** 4 | **Nutrition (per serving):** Calories: 300 | Protein: 4 g | Fat: 12 g | Carbs: 42 g

Ingredients:

- 3 cups mixed berries (fresh or frozen)
- 2 tbsp maple syrup
- ½ cup rolled oats
- ¼ cup almond flour
- 2 tbsp coconut oil, melted
- 1 tsp cinnamon

Instructions:

1. Preheat oven to 375°F (190°C).
2. Toss berries with 1 tbsp maple syrup and place in a baking dish.
3. Mix oats, almond flour, coconut oil, cinnamon, and remaining maple syrup; sprinkle over berries.
4. Bake 25–30 minutes until topping is golden. Serve warm.

Lemon Cashew Tart

Prep Time: 20 min | **Chill Time:** 2 hours | **Servings:** 6 | **Nutrition (per serving):** Calories: 280 | Protein: 5 g | Fat: 18 g | Carbs: 24 g

Ingredients:

- **Crust:** 1 cup almonds, ½ cup dates, pinch of salt
- **Filling:** 1 cup cashews, soaked 4 hours
- ¼ cup lemon juice

- 3 tbsp maple syrup
- 1 tsp vanilla extract

Instructions:

1. Blend almonds, dates, and salt for crust. Press into tart pan.
2. Blend-soaked cashews with lemon juice, maple syrup, and vanilla for filling.
3. Pour filling over crust and chill 2 hours until firm.
4. Slice and serve.

Hummus & Veggie Wrap

Prep Time: 10 min | **Cook Time:** 0 min | **Servings:** 2 | **Nutrition (per serving):** Calories: 310 | Protein: 10 g | Fat: 12 g | Carbs: 42 g

Ingredients:

- 2 large whole-grain tortillas
- ½ cup hummus
- 1 cup mixed greens
- ½ cup shredded carrots
- ½ cucumber, sliced
- ¼ red bell pepper, sliced

Instructions:

1. Spread hummus evenly on each tortilla.
2. Layer greens, carrots, cucumber, and bell pepper.
3. Roll tightly, slice in half, and serve immediately.

Mediterranean Chickpea Bowl

Prep Time: 15 min | **Cook Time:** 0 min | **Servings:** 2 | **Nutrition (per serving):** Calories: 380 | Protein: 14 g | Fat: 14 g | Carbs: 48 g

Ingredients:

- 1 can chickpeas, drained and rinsed
- 1 cup cherry tomatoes, halved
- ½ cucumber, diced
- ¼ red onion, diced
- 2 tbsp olive oil

- 1 tbsp lemon juice
- 1 tsp dried oregano
- Salt and pepper to taste
- 2 cups cooked brown rice or quinoa

Instructions:

1. In a bowl, combine chickpeas, tomatoes, cucumber, and onion.
2. Drizzle with olive oil and lemon juice, sprinkle oregano, salt, and pepper.
3. Serve over cooked rice or quinoa.

Dinner Recipes

Creamy Coconut Lentil Curry

Prep Time: 10 min | **Cook Time:** 25 min | **Servings:** 4 | **Nutrition (per serving):** Calories: 320 | Protein: 14 g | Fat: 12 g | Carbs: 40 g

Ingredients:

- 1 cup red lentils, rinsed
- 1 tbsp coconut oil
- 1 onion, finely chopped
- 3 garlic cloves, minced
- 1 tbsp ginger, grated
- 1 can (14 oz) coconut milk
- 1 can (14 oz) diced tomatoes
- 1 tsp turmeric
- 1 tsp cumin
- 1 tsp coriander
- ½ tsp chili flakes (optional)
- Salt and pepper to taste
- Fresh cilantro for garnish

Instructions:

1. Heat coconut oil in a pan over medium heat. Sauté onion until soft, 3–4 minutes.
2. Add garlic and ginger; cook 1 minute until fragrant.
3. Stir in turmeric, cumin, coriander, and chili flakes.

4. Add lentils, coconut milk, and tomatoes. Bring to a boil, then simmer 20 minutes, stirring occasionally.

5. Season with salt and pepper. Serve garnished with cilantro.

Stuffed Sweet Potatoes with Chickpeas & Spinach

Prep Time: 10 min | **Cook Time:** 40 min | **Servings:** 4 | **Nutrition (per serving):** Calories: 310 | Protein: 12 g | Fat: 9 g | Carbs: 50 g

Ingredients:

- 4 medium sweet potatoes
- 1 can (15 oz) chickpeas, drained and rinsed
- 2 cups fresh spinach
- 1 tbsp olive oil
- 1 tsp smoked paprika
- ½ tsp garlic powder
- Salt and pepper to taste
- 2 tbsp tahini (optional)

Instructions:

1. Preheat oven to 425°F (220°C). Pierce sweet potatoes with a fork and bake 35–40 minutes until tender.

2. Heat olive oil in a pan, add chickpeas, smoked paprika, garlic powder, salt, and pepper. Cook 5–7 minutes.

3. Add spinach and cook until wilted.

4. Slice baked sweet potatoes open and stuff with chickpea-spinach mixture. Drizzle with tahini if desired.

Creamy Cashew Alfredo Pasta

Prep Time: 10 min | **Cook Time:** 15 min | **Servings:** 4 | **Nutrition (per serving):** Calories: 400 | Protein: 12 g | Fat: 18 g | Carbs: 48 g

Ingredients:

- 12 oz fettuccine or pasta of choice
- 1 cup raw cashews, soaked 2 hours
- 1 cup unsweetened almond milk
- 2 tbsp nutritional yeast
- 2 garlic cloves
- 1 tsp lemon juice
- Salt and pepper to taste
- Fresh parsley for garnish

Instructions:

1. Cook pasta according to package instructions. Drain and set aside.
2. Blend soaked cashews, almond milk, nutritional yeast, garlic, and lemon juice until smooth.
3. Pour sauce into a pan and warm over medium heat, seasoning with salt and pepper.
4. Toss pasta in sauce and garnish with parsley. Serve immediately.

Vegan Stir-Fry with Tempeh

Prep Time: 15 min | **Cook Time:** 15 min | **Servings:** 2 | **Nutrition (per serving):** Calories: 380 | Protein: 22 g | Fat: 16 g | Carbs: 38 g

Ingredients:

- 1 block tempeh, cubed
- 1 tbsp sesame oil
- 1 cup broccoli florets
- 1 red bell pepper, sliced
- 1 carrot, sliced
- 2 tbsp soy sauce or tamari
- 1 tbsp maple syrup
- 1 tsp grated ginger
- 1 garlic clove, minced
- 1 tsp sesame seeds (optional)

Instructions:

1. Heat sesame oil in a pan over medium heat. Add tempeh cubes and cook until golden brown, 5–7 minutes.
2. Add vegetables, garlic, and ginger; sauté 5 minutes.
3. Mix soy sauce and maple syrup; pour over stir-fry and cook 2–3 minutes.
4. Sprinkle with sesame seeds and serve with rice or noodles.

Eggplant & Chickpea Stew

Prep Time: 15 min | **Cook Time:** 30 min | **Servings:** 4 | **Nutrition (per serving):** Calories: 290 | Protein: 11 g | Fat: 10 g | Carbs: 42 g

Ingredients:

- 1 medium eggplant, diced
- 1 can chickpeas, drained
- 1 onion, chopped
- 2 garlic cloves, minced
- 1 can (14 oz) diced tomatoes
- 1 tsp smoked paprika
- 1 tsp cumin
- 1 tbsp olive oil
- Salt and pepper to taste
- Fresh parsley for garnish

Instructions:

1. Heat olive oil in a pot. Sauté onion and garlic 3–4 minutes.
2. Add eggplant, cook 5 minutes.
3. Stir in chickpeas, tomatoes, paprika, cumin, salt, and pepper. Simmer 20 minutes.
4. Serve garnished with parsley.

Vegan Tacos with Black Bean & Corn

Prep Time: 10 min | **Cook Time:** 10 min | **Servings:** 4 | **Nutrition (per serving, 2 tacos):** Calories: 320 | Protein: 12 g | Fat: 10 g | Carbs: 44 g

Ingredients:

- 8 small corn tortillas
- 1 can black beans, drained
- 1 cup corn kernels
- 1 tsp cumin
- 1 tsp chili powder
- Salt and pepper to taste
- ½ avocado, sliced
- Salsa and fresh cilantro for topping

Instructions:

1. Heat black beans, corn, cumin, chili powder, salt, and pepper in a skillet 5–7 minutes.
2. Warm tortillas in a pan.
3. Fill each tortilla with bean-corn mixture. Top with avocado, salsa, and cilantro.

Snacks & Sides Recipes

Roasted Spiced Chickpeas

Prep Time: 5 min | **Cook Time:** 25 min | **Servings:** 4 | **Nutrition (per serving):** Calories: 180 | Protein: 8 g | Fat: 5 g | Carbs: 28 g

Ingredients:

- 1 can chickpeas, drained and rinsed
- 1 tbsp olive oil
- 1 tsp smoked paprika
- ½ tsp garlic powder
- ½ tsp cumin
- Salt and pepper to taste

Instructions:

1. Preheat oven to 400°F (200°C).
2. Toss chickpeas with olive oil, smoked paprika, garlic powder, cumin, salt, and pepper.
3. Spread on a baking sheet and roast 20–25 minutes, shaking halfway through, until crispy.
4. Serve warm or at room temperature as a crunchy snack.

Vegan Cheese Dip with Veggies

Prep Time: 10 min | **Cook Time:** 10 min | **Servings:** 4 | **Nutrition (per serving):** Calories: 150 | Protein: 6 g | Fat: 9 g | Carbs: 12 g

Ingredients:

- 1 cup raw cashews, soaked 2 hours
- ½ cup unsweetened almond milk
- 2 tbsp nutritional yeast
- 1 tsp lemon juice
- ½ tsp garlic powder
- Salt and pepper to taste
- Fresh veggies for dipping (carrots, cucumber, bell pepper)

Instructions:

1. Blend cashews, almond milk, nutritional yeast, lemon juice, garlic powder, salt, and pepper until smooth.
2. Warm slightly in a pan if desired.
3. Serve with fresh vegetable sticks for dipping.

Veggie Spring Rolls

Prep Time: 15 min | **Cook Time:** 0 min | **Servings:** 4 | **Nutrition (per serving, 2 rolls):** Calories: 140 | Protein: 4 g | Fat: 3 g | Carbs: 26 g

Ingredients:

- 8 rice paper wrappers
- 1 cup shredded cabbage
- 1 carrot, julienned
- ½ cucumber, julienned

- ½ avocado, sliced
- Fresh mint and cilantro leaves
- Soy sauce or peanut sauce for dipping

Instructions:

1. Soak one rice paper wrapper in warm water until soft.
2. Place vegetables and herbs in the center, fold in sides, and roll tightly.
3. Repeat with remaining wrappers and filling.
4. Serve with soy or peanut dipping sauce.

Spiced Nuts

Prep Time: 5 min | **Cook Time:** 15 min | **Servings:** 4 | **Nutrition (per serving):** Calories: 200 | Protein: 5 g | Fat: 18 g | Carbs: 8 g

Ingredients:

- 2 cups mixed nuts (almonds, cashews, pecans)
- 1 tbsp olive oil or maple syrup
- 1 tsp smoked paprika
- ½ tsp cinnamon
- ½ tsp salt

Instructions:

1. Preheat oven to 350°F (175°C).
2. Toss nuts with olive oil or maple syrup, smoked paprika, cinnamon, and salt.
3. Spread on a baking sheet and roast 12–15 minutes, stirring halfway.

4. Cool slightly and enjoy as a healthy snack.

🍲 Main Dishes/Dinner

Chickpea & Quinoa Power Bowl

Ingredients:

- 1 cup cooked quinoa
- 1 cup roasted chickpeas (seasoned with paprika + garlic)
- 1 cup steamed broccoli
- ½ avocado, sliced
- Tahini dressing (2 Tbsp tahini, lemon juice, garlic, water to thin)

Instructions:

1. Layer quinoa, chickpeas, broccoli, and avocado in a bowl.
2. Drizzle with tahini dressing.

✨ *Health Tip:* Combines plant protein, healthy fats, and fiber for a balanced meal.

Sweet Potato & Black Bean Tacos

Ingredients:

- 2 medium sweet potatoes, roasted and cubed
- 1 cup black beans (cooked)
- ½ cup corn kernels
- 6 small corn tortillas
- Salsa + cilantro for topping

Instructions:

1. Roast sweet potato cubes at 400°F for 25 minutes.
2. Warm tortillas and fill with sweet potatoes, beans, and corn.
3. Top with salsa and cilantro.

✨ *Health Tip:* A fiber-packed twist on tacos with natural sweetness from sweet potatoes.

Lentil and Vegetable Curry

Ingredients:

- 1 cup red lentils
- 1 onion, diced
- 2 cloves garlic, minced
- 1 can coconut milk
- 2 cups mixed vegetables (carrots, peas, spinach)
- 2 Tbsp curry powder
- Salt to taste

Instructions:

1. Sauté onion and garlic.
2. Add curry powder, lentils, coconut milk, and 2 cups water.
3. Simmer until lentils are soft; stir in vegetables.

✨ *Health Tip:* Lentils provide protein and iron, making this a comforting, healing meal.

Creamy Coconut Lentil Curry

Prep Time: 10 min | **Cook Time:** 25 min | **Servings:** 4

Ingredients:

- 1 cup red lentils, rinsed
- 1 tbsp coconut oil
- 1 onion, finely chopped
- 3 garlic cloves, minced
- 1 tbsp ginger, grated
- 1 can (14 oz) coconut milk
- 1 can (14 oz) diced tomatoes
- 1 tsp turmeric
- 1 tsp cumin
- 1 tsp coriander
- ½ tsp chili flakes (optional)
- Salt and pepper to taste
- Fresh cilantro for garnish

Instructions:

1. Heat coconut oil in a large pan over medium heat. Sauté onion until soft, 3–4 minutes.
2. Add garlic and ginger; cook for 1 minute until fragrant.
3. Stir in turmeric, cumin, coriander, and chili flakes.
4. Add lentils, coconut milk, and tomatoes. Bring to a boil, then reduce heat and simmer 20 minutes, stirring occasionally.
5. Season with salt and pepper. Serve hot, garnished with fresh cilantro.

Quinoa & Roasted Veggie Buddha Bowl

Prep Time: 15 min | **Cook Time:** 30 min | **Servings:** 2

Ingredients:

- 1 cup quinoa
- 2 cups water or vegetable broth
- 1 zucchini, sliced
- 1 red bell pepper, chopped
- 1 cup broccoli florets
- 2 tbsp olive oil
- 1 tsp smoked paprika
- Salt and pepper to taste
- ¼ cup tahini
- 2 tbsp lemon juice
- 1 tbsp maple syrup
- Water to thin

Instructions:

1. Preheat oven to 400°F (200°C). Toss zucchini, bell pepper, and broccoli with olive oil, smoked paprika, salt, and pepper. Roast for 20–25 minutes.
2. Rinse quinoa and cook with water or broth according to package instructions.
3. Whisk tahini, lemon juice, maple syrup, and enough water to make a smooth dressing.
4. Serve quinoa in bowls topped with roasted veggies and drizzle with tahini dressing.

Chickpea & Spinach Stuffed Sweet Potatoes

Prep Time: 10 min | **Cook Time:** 40 min | **Servings:** 4

Ingredients:

- 4 medium sweet potatoes
- 1 can (15 oz) chickpeas, drained and rinsed
- 2 cups fresh spinach
- 1 tbsp olive oil
- 1 tsp smoked paprika
- ½ tsp garlic powder
- Salt and pepper to taste
- 2 tbsp tahini (optional)

Instructions:

1. Preheat oven to 425°F (220°C). Pierce sweet potatoes with a fork and bake 35–40 minutes until tender.
2. While potatoes bake, heat olive oil in a pan, add chickpeas, smoked paprika, garlic powder, salt, and pepper. Cook 5–7 minutes.
3. Add spinach and cook until wilted.
4. Slice baked sweet potatoes open and stuff with chickpea-spinach mixture. Drizzle with tahini if desired.

✨ *Health Tip:* Lentils provide protein and iron, making this a comforting, healing meal.

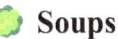 Soups & Salads

Creamy Butternut Squash Soup

Ingredients:

- 1 medium butternut squash, peeled and cubed
- 1 onion, chopped
- 2 cloves garlic
- 3 cups vegetable broth
- 1 tsp thyme
- 1 cup coconut milk

Instructions:

1. Roast squash at 400°F until tender.
2. Sauté onion and garlic, add squash, broth, and thyme.
3. Blend until smooth; stir in coconut milk.

✦ *Health Tip:* A warming, immune-boosting soup rich in vitamin

Mediterranean Kale Salad

Ingredients:

- 3 cups kale, chopped
- ½ cup cherry tomatoes
- ¼ cup olives
- ¼ cup chickpeas

- Lemon-tahini dressing

Instructions:
1. Massage kale with a little olive oil.
2. Toss with tomatoes, olives, chickpeas, and dressing.

✨ *Health Tip:* **Massaging kale reduces bitterness and makes nutrients easier to absorb.**

🍏 Snacks

Roasted Spiced Chickpeas

Ingredients:

- 1 can chickpeas, drained and dried
- 1 Tbsp olive oil
- 1 tsp paprika
- ½ tsp garlic powder
- ½ tsp cumin

Instructions:

1. Toss chickpeas with oil and spices.
2. Roast at 400°F for 25–30 minutes.

✨ *Health Tip:* Crunchy, protein-packed snack to replace chips.

Hummus with Veggie Sticks

Ingredients:

- 1 can chickpeas
- 2 Tbsp tahini
- 2 cloves garlic
- Juice of 1 lemon
- Olive oil + salt

Instructions:

1. Blend chickpeas, tahini, garlic, and lemon.
2. Add olive oil until creamy.
3. Serve with cucumber, carrot, and celery sticks.

✨ *Health Tip:* Great source of fiber and healthy fats.

🥤 Smoothies & Drinks

Smoothie – Green Glow Smoothie

Ingredients:

- 2 cups spinach
- 1 banana
- 1 cup frozen mango
- 1 cup unsweetened oat milk
- 1 Tbsp flaxseeds

Instructions:

1. Blend all ingredients until smooth.
2. Pour into a glass and enjoy immediately.

Green Glow Smoothie

Ingredients:

- 2 cups spinach
- 1 banana
- 1 cup frozen mango
- 1 cup oat milk
- 1 Tbsp flaxseeds

Instructions:

1. Blend until smooth and creamy.

✨ *Health Tip:* Boosts digestion and skin health.

Berry Protein Shake

Ingredients:

- 1 cup mixed berries (frozen)
- 1 scoop plant protein powder
- 1 cup soy milk
- 1 Tbsp almond butter

Instructions:

1. Blend all ingredients until smooth.

✨ *Health Tip:* Perfect post-workout recovery shake.

◆ Desserts

Chocolaté Avocado Mousse

Ingrédients:

- 2 ripe avocados
- ¼ cup cocoa powder
- ¼ cup maple syrup
- 1 tsp vanilla extract
- Pinch of sea salt

Instructions:

1. Blend until creamy.
2. Chill before serving.

✨ *Health Tip:* Healthy fats + antioxidants make this dessert guilt-free.

Coconut Chia Pudding

Ingredients:

- 3 Tbsp chia seeds
- 1 cup coconut milk
- 1 Tbsp maple syrup
- ½ tsp vanilla extract

Instructions:

1. Mix all ingredients in a jar.

2. Refrigerate overnight.
3. Top with fruit before serving.

✨ *Health Tip:* High in omega-3s and fiber, excellent for digestion.

Baked Cinnamon Apples

Ingredients:

- 2 apples, cored and sliced
- 1 tsp cinnamon
- 1 tsp maple syrup
- ¼ cup walnuts

Instructions:

1. Place apples in a baking dish.
2. Sprinkle with cinnamon, maple syrup, and walnuts.
3. Bake at 375°F for 20 minutes.

✨ *Health Tip:* A naturally sweet, antioxidant-rich treat.

Chocolate Avocado Mousse

Prep Time: 10 min | **Chill Time:** 1 hour | **Servings:** 4

Ingredients:

- 2 ripe avocados
- ¼ cup cocoa powder

- ¼ cup maple syrup (adjust to taste)
- 1 tsp vanilla extract
- Pinch of salt
- Fresh berries for topping

Instructions:

1. Blend avocados, cocoa powder, maple syrup, vanilla, and salt until creamy and smooth.
2. Chill in the refrigerator for at least 1 hour.
3. Serve in bowls or glasses topped with fresh berries.

🧁 Fluffy Vegan Banana Bread

Ingredients

- 3 ripe bananas, mashed
- ½ cup coconut sugar
- ¼ cup coconut oil, melted
- 1 tsp vanilla extract
- 1 ½ cups whole wheat flour
- 1 tsp baking soda
- ½ tsp salt
- ½ tsp cinnamon

Instructions

1. Preheat oven to 350°F (175°C).
2. Mix bananas, sugar, oil, and vanilla.
3. In a separate bowl, whisk flour, baking soda, salt, and cinnamon.
4. Combine wet and dry, pour into loaf pan.
5. Bake 45–50 minutes. Cool before slicing.

◆ Double Chocolate Vegan Brownies

Ingredients

- 1 cup oat flour
- ½ cup cocoa powder
- ½ cup almond butter
- ½ cup maple syrup
- 1 tsp vanilla extract
- ½ tsp baking soda
- ½ cup dairy-free chocolate chips

Instructions

1. Preheat oven to 350°F. Line a baking pan.
2. Mix all ingredients until smooth.
3. Fold in chocolate chips.
4. Bake for 25–30 minutes.
5. Let cool completely before

🍪 Classic Chewy Chocolate Chip Cookies

Ingredients

- 1 cup coconut sugar (or brown sugar)
- ½ cup coconut oil, softened
- ¼ cup almond milk
- 1 tbsp flaxseed meal + 3 tbsp water (flax egg)
- 1 tsp vanilla extract
- 1 ½ cups all-purpose flour
- ½ tsp baking soda
- ½ tsp baking powder
- ½ tsp salt
- 1 cup dairy

🌱 Reflections: A Journey of Nourishment and Purpose

As you reach the end of this book, know that your journey is just beginning. Every recipe you've explored, every ingredient you've discovered, and every mindful choice you've made is a step toward a more compassionate, vibrant, and balanced life.

Veganism is not simply a diet it's a movement of love. It's an invitation to live with intention, to care deeply for your body, to honor the Earth, and to extend kindness to all living beings. Each meal becomes an act of healing for yourself, for others, and for the world we share. Through nourishing your body with plants, you also nourish your spirit with peace. You cultivate energy that uplifts not only your own life but also the lives of those around you. With every plant-based meal, you make a statement of compassion, sustainability, and self-respect.

"When we choose to live consciously, we become the change we wish to see. " Whether you started this journey for your health, for the animals, or for the planet your choice matters. Your commitment is powerful. And your example has the potential to inspire others to live with greater awareness, empathy, and joy.

As you continue cooking, experimenting, and learning, remember that veganism is a path of growth one filled with discovery, flavor, and love. May your kitchen be a sanctuary of creativity and your meals a celebration of life itself.

Thank you for choosing kindness. Thank you for choosing life. And thank you for allowing this book to be part of your journey toward a healthier, more compassionate world.

With gratitude and light,
Dr. Sandra Johnson
Author & Advocate for Wellness, Compassion, and Conscious Living

🌿 Faith & Compassion: The Heart of Vegan Living

🌸 The Spiritual Foundation of Compassion

Faith and compassion are deeply connected both teach us to live with empathy, kindness, and gratitude. Many spiritual paths emphasize the sacredness of life and the importance of caring for creation. Veganism naturally aligns with these values by extending compassion beyond humans to animals, the environment, and all living things.

When we choose veganism, we are making a conscious decision to live in harmony with the principles of love and mercy that our faith calls us to embody.
It's a daily act of reverence a way to honor the divine through the care we give to ourselves and the world around us.

🌸 Faith as Guidance in Daily Choices

Faith often calls us to walk in love and integrity. Choosing veganism can be seen as a *spiritual practice* one that allows us to live our beliefs rather than just speak them.
Each meal becomes a prayer of gratitude, a symbol of peace, and a reflection of our inner values.

You might say a short reflection before meals, such as:

"May this food nourish my body, uplift my spirit, and reflect the love and compassion that guide my heart."

This brings awareness, gratitude, and sacredness into the act of eating.

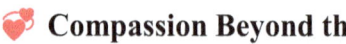 **Compassion Beyond the Plate**

Compassion is more than feeling sorry for others it's *love in action*. When you live compassionately, you recognize the divine spark in every being.
Veganism becomes a form of active compassion a way of saying:

"Your life matters. Your suffering matters. I choose peace."

It's also about self-compassion. Many people come to veganism not only to help animals but also to *heal themselves* physically, mentally, and spiritually. The practice of compassion begins with how we treat our own bodies and souls.

🌍 The Ripple Effect of Kindness

A compassionate lifestyle creates ripples of goodness far beyond what we can see.
When we choose kindness over convenience, we reduce harm to animals, protect the planet, and inspire others to do the same.
Faith reminds us that even small acts of love carry great power.
Each vegan choice a meal, a word, a gesture becomes a seed of healing sown into the world.

✨ Living Faithfully, Living Kindly

True faith shines in how we live. It is expressed through patience, forgiveness, and empathy not only toward people but all of creation. When we live in alignment with our faith and compassion, our bodies become temples of peace, our food becomes blessings, and our actions become prayers.

Affirmation:

"I walk in love. I live with compassion. My choices are reflections of my faith."

🌼 Reflection Questions

To make this interactive, you could include a short reflection page:

- How does my faith influence the way I treat living beings?
- In what ways can I show more compassion to myself, to others, and to animals?
- What does living kindly mean to me?

- How can I bring gratitude and prayerfulness into my meals?

Faith and compassion together create a way of life that feeds the soul. Veganism, at its essence, is love made visible it's choosing peace on your plate and in your heart.
It reminds us that living with faith means *acting with love*, and living with compassion means *honoring life in all its forms.*

🌿 Faith & Compassion: The Heartbeat of a Vegan Life

🌸 Faith as the Root of Conscious Living

Faith is more than a belief it's a way of life, a daily walk of trust, gratitude, and love.
For many, faith calls us to live with purpose and to honor the sacredness of all creation. It reminds us that our actions, no matter how small, carry meaning.
Choosing veganism can be one of the purest expressions of faith a way of practicing love and mercy toward every living being, just as many spiritual teachings instruct.

Whether one's faith is rooted in Christianity, spirituality, mindfulness, or a universal belief in goodness, the message remains the same:

Love one another. Be kind. Do no harm.

When we apply that principle beyond ourselves to animals, nature, and the planet our faith becomes living, breathing compassion.

😊 Compassion as a Divine Expression

Compassion is the purest form of love in action. It is empathy made visible the desire to ease suffering wherever we encounter it.
Faith inspires compassion, and compassion sustains faith. Together, they become the moral and spiritual compass that guides a vegan lifestyle.

Each vegan choice becomes a sacred act not out of obligation, but out of devotion.
When we choose foods that do not cause harm, we align our inner peace with the outer world.
We begin to live in harmony with the divine rhythm of creation, honoring life as sacred.

💖 The Connection Between Body, Spirit, and Compassion

Many faith traditions teach that the body is a temple — a vessel for divine energy.
When we nourish our bodies with pure, life-giving foods, we treat this temple with respect. Plant-based foods bring vitality, clarity, and healing not only to the body but also to the soul.

Veganism becomes an act of spiritual discipline a practice that brings mindfulness to eating, gratitude to nourishment, and reverence to life. Every meal becomes a quiet moment of worship a reminder that gratitude and compassion can be practiced through simple, daily choices.

You might say:

"Thank you, Earth, for this nourishment. Thank you, Creator, for the gift of life. May I live in harmony with all beings."

Faith Calls Us to Be Stewards of Creation

Many sacred teachings remind us that we are caretakers of the Earth. Faith invites us to act responsibly to protect what has been entrusted to us, not exploit it.
Veganism embodies that stewardship by reducing harm to animals, conserving natural resources, and helping heal our planet.

By embracing a plant-based lifestyle, we fulfill our duty to care for the Earth and its inhabitants.
It becomes a form of worship living with gratitude for creation and using our choices to honor it.

"Compassion is not only what we feel; it's what we *do* with what we feel."

🌱 Forgiveness, Grace, and Growth

Faith also teaches forgiveness for others and for ourselves.
Not everyone begins their journey perfectly. Some people stumble, struggle, or return to old habits.
That's okay. Compassion includes *self-compassion*.

Forgive yourself for what you didn't know before.
Celebrate every step toward kindness, no matter how small.
Every day offers a new opportunity to live with more love, more awareness, and more peace.

Affirmation:

"I am growing in compassion. My journey is guided by faith, not perfection."

🌻 Faith Unites All Living Beings

Faith and compassion remind us of our connection that all life is intertwined.
When one being suffers, creation suffers. When we live kindly, we bring healing not only to animals and the planet but to our own hearts.

This awareness brings a sense of sacred unity that we are all part of something greater, a divine web of life that thrives on love and balance.
Veganism honors that unity.

It says, *"Your life is sacred. Your pain matters. I choose peace."*

🌈 Faith, Joy, and Gratitude

Living compassionately through faith isn't about deprivation it's about abundance.
It's about tasting the richness of life without harm.
Faith fills the heart with joy, and compassion gives that joy purpose.

Each meal becomes a moment to express gratitude:

- Gratitude for the Earth's fruits and grains.
- Gratitude for health and nourishment.
- Gratitude for the opportunity to live in love and peace.

This is the spiritual beauty of veganism not just changing what's on the plate, but transforming what's in the heart.

Reflection for the Soul

Invite readers to pause and journal:

1. How does my faith inspire compassion in my daily life?
2. What does it mean for me to "live kindly"?
3. How can I express gratitude through the way I eat, live, and treat others?
4. In what ways do my actions honor my faith and values?
5. How can I show mercy not just to others, but to myself?

✨ Reflection

Faith is love, and compassion is its voice.
When faith leads us toward kindness, and kindness leads us toward action, we begin to embody the deepest truth of all spiritual paths that love is the foundation of everything.

To live vegan is to live faithfully.

It's to say with every choice, *"I honor life. I choose peace. I walk with love."*
And in doing so, you create a legacy of healing for the Earth, for others, and for your own soul.

🌍 Advocacy & Community: Building a World Rooted in Compassion

🌿 The Power of Collective Change

Veganism begins with one person one heart, one choice, one meal. But when millions of people make that same choice, it becomes a *movement*. Advocacy and community give veganism its voice they transform private conviction into public compassion.

We live in a world where food connects us, where culture and conversation grow around the table. Every time we share a vegan meal, story, or idea, we are planting seeds of awareness. Advocacy is not about preaching; it's about *inspiring*. It's about showing others the beauty, flavor, and kindness that come from living compassionately.

"When you share from love, you awaken love in others."

🤝 Community: The Heartbeat of the Movement

Community is where strength multiplies. It reminds us that we are not alone — that others share our hope for a kinder, healthier, and more sustainable world.

A vegan community can be local or global from a small support group to online platforms where people connect, share recipes, and uplift one another.

Building community means:

- Supporting local vegan restaurants, farmers, and small businesses.
- Volunteering at animal sanctuaries or plant-based education centers.
- Hosting potlucks, wellness workshops, or plant-based cooking classes.
- Sharing vegan meals with friends and family to open loving conversations.

These moments bring people together, creating bonds rooted in compassion and common purpose.

"The table of kindness has room for everyone."

💚 Advocacy with Grace and Respect

Advocacy doesn't mean argument it means *gentle influence*. True advocacy is leading by example, showing others through your actions how fulfilling and joyful vegan living can be.

When we advocate with patience, kindness, and understanding, we reflect the very values veganism stands for.
Instead of focusing on judgment, we focus on education and encouragement.

Effective advocacy can take many forms:

- **Storytelling:** Sharing your journey what inspired you, what challenges you overcame, how your health and spirit improved.
- **Education:** Providing factual, compassionate information about plant-based nutrition, environmental impact, or animal welfare.
- **Empathy:** Listening to others' perspectives without criticism and responding with care and clarity.

"Be the example of the change you wish to see not by demand, but by demonstration."

❀ Creating Safe Spaces for Dialogue

True community grows in safe, welcoming spaces. As advocates, we create environments where people can explore veganism without fear of judgment or guilt.
We meet people where they are, understanding that change is a journey.

In faith-based or family-centered settings, gentle conversations about compassion and stewardship can bridge understanding. Offering a delicious vegan meal or sharing a personal testimony often speaks louder than words.
When people feel loved and accepted, they are more open to transformation.

"Compassion opens doors that judgment keeps closed."

🌱 Global Impact, Local Action

While veganism has global benefits reducing deforestation, conserving water, and protecting wildlife the movement grows strongest through *local action*.
Small acts of service within our communities' ripple outward into the world.

Ways to make a difference locally:

- Organize community clean-ups, food drives, or wellness fairs with a vegan message.
- Partner with schools or youth programs to teach plant-based nutrition.
- Support social justice movements that align with compassion and sustainability.
- Collaborate with churches, mosques, temples, or civic groups to promote stewardship of creation.

Each community effort embodies the belief that compassion belongs in every space spiritual, cultural, and social.

🐾 Speaking for the Voiceless

At the heart of vegan advocacy is a voice for those who cannot speak — animals.
Advocacy gives life to empathy, urging the world to recognize that all beings share the capacity for love, pain, and connection.

We do not need to shock or shame people to awaken compassion. We can teach through beauty through vibrant food, loving action, and peaceful presence.
When we share stories of rescued animals, environmental healing, or personal transformation, we remind people that kindness is not extreme it is *our natural state*.

"To advocate for the voiceless is to speak the language of the soul."

🌈 Unity Through Compassion

Vegan advocacy isn't about dividing the world into "us" and "them." It's about uniting people through love and understanding. Compassion transcends differences faith, culture, age, or background.
We are all connected through the Earth that sustains us and the universal desire to live in peace.

When communities come together around compassion, they create hope. They become examples of love in action the kind of love that heals, restores, and uplifts humanity as a whole.

💖 Encouraging the Next Generation

One of the most powerful forms of advocacy is *inspiring youth*. Teaching children empathy toward animals, environmental care, and healthy eating builds a generation of mindful, compassionate leaders. Let them see that veganism isn't about restriction it's about abundance, creativity, and respect for life.

When children understand where their food comes from, they naturally develop empathy and awareness. By empowering the next generation, we shape a future grounded in love.

🌻 Reflection and Action

1. How can I use my voice to inspire compassion in others?
2. What can I do within my community to promote kindness and awareness?
3. How can I lead with love rather than judgment?
4. What causes align with my values that I can support or create?
5. How can I help others see veganism as a joyful, faith-aligned, and healing way of life?

🌱 Vegan Affirmations for Mind, Body & Spirit

💚 Faith & Compassion

1. "I walk in love, live in kindness, and eat in peace."
2. "My choices honor creation and reflect the compassion in my heart."
3. "I am guided by faith, strengthened by love, and grounded in gratitude."
4. "Each meal I prepare is an act of reverence for all life."
5. "Through compassion, I become a vessel of divine love."
6. "My plate reflects my prayers peaceful, kind, and full of grace."
7. "As I nourish my body with plants, I nourish my soul with purpose."
8. "I am a caretaker of life, walking gently upon the Earth."

❀ Health, Healing & Wholeness

1. "I feed my body foods that bring healing, balance, and light."
2. "With every plant-based meal, I strengthen my health and my heart."
3. "I am grateful for the energy and clarity that nature provides."
4. "Vibrant foods create a vibrant life."
5. "What I eat becomes part of who I am today, I choose life."
6. "I honor my body as a temple by nourishing it with kindness."
7. "My body thrives on the purity of plants and the power of love."
8. "I am becoming healthier, happier, and more peaceful every day."

🌿 Mindfulness & Gratitude

1. "Each bite is a moment of gratitude for the earth's generosity."
2. "I eat mindfully, with love for all who made this meal possible."
3. "Peace begins with what I place on my plate."
4. "I am thankful for the beauty and abundance of nature."
5. "I live each day with awareness, kindness, and appreciation."
6. "My food choices are a reflection of my respect for life."
7. "In stillness and gratitude, I find nourishment for my soul."
8. "I live each moment in harmony with the world around me."

🌻 Advocacy & Community

1. "My voice carries love, not judgment."
2. "I lead by example gently, joyfully, and authentically."
3. "I use my light to inspire others to live kindly."
4. "Community grows through compassion and shared purpose."
5. "Every small act of kindness creates ripples of change."
6. "I am part of a global family rooted in love for all beings."
7. "Through unity and empathy, we create a kinder world."
8. "My advocacy is my prayer my compassion is my strength."

✨ Spiritual Growth & Self-Compassion

1. "I release guilt and embrace grace growth is a journey, not perfection."
2. "I forgive myself for the past and celebrate the progress of today."
3. "I walk with faith, I act with kindness, I live with peace."
4. "Every compassionate choice strengthens my spirit."
5. "I am aligned with love my heart, my actions, and my faith."
6. "I honor my path and trust divine timing in all things."
7. "I am evolving into a more loving and conscious version of myself."
8. "Kindness toward others begins with kindness toward myself."

🌺 Inspirational Vegan Quotes

🌿 On Compassion & Kindness

1. "Until we extend our circle of compassion to all living things, humanity will not find peace." - *Albert Schweitzer*
2. "The greatness of a nation and its moral progress can be judged by the way its animals are treated." -*Mahatma Gandhi*
3. "Kindness is the language which the deaf can hear and the blind can see." - *Mark Twain*
4. "Veganism is not a sacrifice; it is a joy that comes from living your values." -*Colleen Patrick-Goudreau*
5. "Be kind to every kind not just mankind." -*Unknown*
6. "Our lives begin to end the day we become silent about things that matter." -*Martin Luther King Jr.*
7. "To care for others human or animal is the highest expression of our humanity." - *Unknown*

🌸 On Faith & Purpose

1. "Faith is not just what we believe; it's how we live what we believe." - *Unknown*
2. "When you live from love, every act becomes a prayer." *-Dr. Sandra Johnson*
3. "Compassion is the truest reflection of divine grace." *- Unknown*
4. "We are stewards, not owners, of this Earth called to protect, not exploit." - *Inspired by Psalm 24:1*
5. "Living vegan is living faithfully with reverence for life and respect for creation." - *Unknown*

🌻 On Health & Healing

1. "Let food be thy medicine and medicine be thy food."
   - *Hippocrates*
2. "What you eat literally becomes you. Choose wisely, choose kindly." - *Unknown*
3. "Healing begins the moment you honor your body as sacred." -*Unknown*
4. "A plant-based life isn't about restriction it's about restoration." -*Unknown*

🌈 On Community & Change

1. "Never doubt that a small group of thoughtful, committed citizens can change the world." — *Margaret Mead*
2. "Together we rise by lifting others." — *Robert Ingersoll*
3. "Community is the heart of change where compassion becomes action." — *Unknown*
4. "Every conversation rooted in kindness becomes a seed of transformation." — *Unknown*

🌿 On Gratitude & Inner Peace

1. "Gratitude turns every meal into a feast of blessings."
   -*Unknown*
2. "Peace doesn't start in the world it starts on our plate."
   - *Unknown*
3. "When you eat with mindfulness, you feed your spirit as much as your body." -*Thich Nhat Hanh*
4. "The more thankful you are, the more peaceful you become."
   -Unknown

🍃 "Veganism is love in action faith made visible through compassion." - *Dr. Sandra Johnson*

1. "Every plant-based choice is a step toward healing for you and for the world." - *Dr. Sandra Johnson*
2. "To live kindly is to live courageously choosing peace even when the world does not." -*Dr. Sandra Johnson*
3. "Compassion on your plate reflects compassion in your soul." - *Dr. Sandra Johnson*
4. "The most powerful transformation begins with a single kind choice." -*Dr. Sandra Johnson*
5. "You don't have to change the whole world just change what's on your plate, and the world begins to change with you."
   -*Dr. Sandra Johnson*

☀ Closing Inspiration

Community is the vessel through which compassion grows, and advocacy is the voice that carries it forward.
When we come together in love and purpose, we transform the world not by force, but by example.
Veganism reminds us that faith without compassion is incomplete, and compassion without action is silent.

So, speak gently, act boldly, and live lovingly.
Let your life be your message a living testament that one person, one meal, one act of kindness *can change everything.*

"When we advocate with love, we don't just change minds we awaken hearts."

A Call to Action

As you close this book, I invite you to do one thing: **take action today.**

- Try one new plant-based recipe tonight.
- Plan your meals for the week ahead.
- Share your "why" with a friend or family member.
- Commit to your next 30 days not perfectly, but intentionally.

Don't wait for the perfect time. The perfect time is *now.*

Final Words: Becoming Fully Alive

Food is more than fuel it's a daily chance to choose life. By choosing plants, you're choosing vitality, longevity, and alignment. You're choosing a path of energy instead of fatigue, clarity instead of fog, growth instead of decline.

This journey isn't about restriction. It's about expansion. More flavors. More health. More possibility. More life.

You hold the power one plate, one choice, one day at a time. And with each choice, you are writing a new story for your body, your mind, and your future.

So, step forward. Live the story. Thrive on plants.

When I look back at where I started "feeling exhausted, carrying extra weight, and worried about my health" I can hardly believe the difference now. Choosing to go vegan for my health wasn't always easy, but it was one of the most powerful decisions I've ever made.

What began as a 30-day experiment has become a lifestyle that feels natural, energizing, and aligned with who I want to be. Along the way, I've learned that this journey is about so much more than food. It's about self-respect. It's about listening to your body. It's about realizing that every meal is a chance to choose life and health.

This Is Your Journey Too

If there's one thing I want you to take away from this book, it's this: **you are capable of change.**

You don't need to do it perfectly. You don't need to have it all figured out. All you need to do is begin one choice, one meal, one day at a time.

When I felt like giving up, I reminded myself of my "why." For me, that was wanting to avoid medication, have more energy for my quality of life, and feel proud of the person I saw in the mirror". Hold onto your "why." Let it guide you when challenges come.

Reader Reflection

Take a few moments to reflect on what this journey has meant to you. Use the prompts below to capture your personal transformation and insights from embracing a vegan lifestyle.

Living vegan is an act of intention it's choosing peace in small, daily ways.
Every meal, every product, every purchase is a statement of love for yourself, the planet, and all living beings.

"Veganism is not perfection it's progression, compassion, and faith in action."

1. What inspired you to begin your vegan journey?

2. How has your relationship with food changed since embracing plant-based eating?

3. What are three words that describe how veganism makes you feel?

4. How can you inspire others to live with more compassion and mindfulness?

5. What goals do you have for continuing your vegan journey?

www.ingramcontent.com/pod-product-compliance
Lightning Source LLC
Chambersburg PA
CBHW070806230426
43663CB00017B/2512